External Ocular Tumors

External Ocular Tumors

A Clinicopathologic Study of 300 Cases

Textbook and Atlas

By Knud Bech and Ove Aksel Jensen

116 Figures, 4 Color-Plates, 7 Tables

1978

W. B. Saunders Company
Philadelphia · London · Toronto

Georg Thieme Publishers Stuttgart

Authors

Knud Bech, M.D., Eye Department, Frederiksberg Hospital,
DK-2000 Copenhagen F, Denmark

Ove Aksel Jensen, M.D., Eye Pathology Institute, University of Copenhagen,
Frederik V's Vej 11, DK-2100 Copenhagen Ø, Denmark

© 1978. Georg Thieme Verlag, Herdweg 63, P.O.B. 732, D-7000 Stuttgart – Printed in Germany by
Grammlich, Pliezhausen

ISBN 3-13-559301-0

English edition co-published 1978 by W.B. Saunders Company, Philadelphia, London, Toronto
and Georg Thieme Verlag, Stuttgart

ISBN: 0-7216-1613-5 (W.B. Saunders)
LCCCN: 77-95076 (W.B. Saunders)

Preface

The present publication has been motivated by the difficulty we have experienced over the years in establishing the correct diagnosis of external tumors of the eye. Even experienced clinicians, on the evidence of pathology request forms, have very often erroneously diagnosed such tumors clinically.

Furthermore, we have found that it is important to stress that any tumor or tumor-like lesion, even the smallest and apparently completely benign lesion, should be examined histopathologically since it may turn out to be malignant. Again, we wished to give the practicing ophthalmologist an opportunity to compare the clinical and histopathological pictures.

For this reason, the illustrations are arranged in groups; the clinical picture is followed generally by a survey of the microscopic section and then by higher magnifications. We have tried to demonstrate the clinical appearance of the tumor in an appropriate size and surrounded by the relevant structures so that the observer will have a natural impression of the tumor and its localization − as if he were sitting in front of the patient inspecting the tumor. We feel that black − white photographs give a satisfactory and often better impression of the clinical appearance and histopathology of the tumor than do color photographs. Such have, therefore, been used only where color is a dominant feature of the tumor.

We have not aimed at a textbook description of the tumors, either clinically or histopathologically, but rather have sought only to indicate the relevant characteristics. We have also not stressed the histopathological classification of the tumors but have assumed our principal purpose to be to deal with the matter from the practitioner's point of view. Dermatologists and radiologists may, perhaps, also derive some help from this monograph.

Please refer to the glossary for definitions of histopathological terms.

We wish to thank the late Professor B. Lavætz, former Chief of the Ophthalmological Department, Rigshospitalet, Tagensvej, for his great interest in this work; we deeply regret that he did not live to see it completed.

Further, we gratefully acknowledge the excellent facilities made available by S. Ry Andersen, Head of the Eye Pathology Institute, University of Copenhagen, and thank him for his helpful criticism.

We are indebted to Hans Fledelius, M. D., Eye Pathology Institute, for reading the manuscript and for his helpful suggestions.

We also acknowledge the skilful technical and secretarial work of the staff of this institute.

The Photographic Department of Rigshospitalet produced the clinical photographs; the staff was always ready to help us, in spite of the heavy burden of routine work.

Practicing ophthalmologists and many ophthalmological departments willingly referred their patients with external tumors to the departments in which we were working, and for this we are grateful.

Last but not least, we are very obliged to the staff of the Radium Center, Finseninstituttet, Copenhagen, for the willingness to collaborate in treating the patients and for the loan of records.

The work was supported by a grant from Statens Lægevidenskabelige Forskningsråd.

January 1978

Knud Bech
Ove Aksel Jensen

Contents

Material and Methods

The study covers 300 consecutive tumors and tumor-like lesions considered as external, i.e., that can be observed by inspecting the conjunctiva and the zones of skin around the eye, particularly the lids and the superciliary region. Tumors in the anterior chamber of the eye are, therefore, not included. This regional limitation may be understood as an expression of the practice employed by the general practitioner in Denmark. Most diseases of the eye and its surroundings are traditionally referred to the ophthalmologist. Since such tumors are usually treated by the practicing ophthalmologist, all ophthalmologists in the island of Zealand were asked in 1965 to refer patients with external tumors to the Eye Department of Rigshospitalet, Tagensvej, Copenhagen. For the most part, this request was complied with. The first 300 patients referred to the department constitute the cases published in this monograph. We, therefore, consider the material to be relevant in relation to the tumors encountered by the ophthalmologist in his daily practice. The material was collected through September 1968.

Each patient was usually examined by one of the authors (KB) and treated surgically by him (cf., special section on treatment). Before treatment, the tumor was photographed and the relevant laboratory examinations made.

The removed tissue was fixed for 24 hours in 4% buffered formaldehyde and prepared routinely according to the usual paraffin technique of the laboratory. The sections were stained with hematoxylin-eosin and according to van Gieson; in some cases, a number of special stains were applied. The histopathological examination was performed by the staff of the laboratory; all sections, however, were re-examined by one of the authors (OAJ). Sections chosen for illustration were stained with hematoxylin-eosin.

All patients with malignant tumors and precancerous lesions as well as a number of other cases were followed up. The follow-up was carried out mainly by means of the records of the Radium Center, Copenhagen. In a number of cases, the patient's own doctor or specialist was consulted. Deceased patients were traced through the Central Card Index for Deaths of the Danish Health Department.

The reason why the material was not divided into tumors of the skin and tumors of the conjunctiva with a separate discussion of each group is that we have attached great importance to a consideration of all the external tumors from a clinical point of view. In the individual sections, however, special features of conjunctival tumors are carefully emphasized; where this is not the case, clinical and histopathological characteristics of skin tumors and conjunctival tumors may be considered identical.

Results

Clinical Findings

Sex and Age

The distribution is shown in Diagram 1. The material comprised 137 males and 163 females. This difference corresponds well to the sex distribution in the Danish population, particularly since more than half the total number of patients were over the age of 50. The percentage of females in the normal population increases with age.

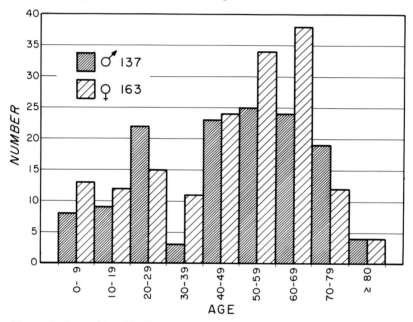

Diagram 1 Sex and Age Distribution

In regard to the frequency of the different tumors within the sex and age groups, it should be mentioned that all cases of **dermoid cysts** (11 cases) were diagnosed in patients under the age of 20. They were three times as frequent in girls as in boys.

Molluscum contagiosum (5 cases) occurred in children and in women under the age of 30. This may, perhaps, be explained by the fact that mothers have the most intimate contact with children.

In regard to the **total** number of nevi (50), no significant sex difference was found. **Nevi of the skin**, however, were twice as frequent in females as in males (cf., section on localization). Regarding the occurrence in the age groups, we found it remarkable that 50% of all nevi in males were removed before the patients reached the age of 30, while in females 75% were removed from patients between the ages of 40 and 70. This may be because many women regard their nevi as "beauty spots" and delay surgical removal until they reach cancerphobic age groups.

Papillomas of the skin and conjunctiva showed an increasing frequency with age and were equally distributed between the sexes. A tendency towards earlier removal was observed in girls; the explanation may well be a cosmetic one such as that mentioned above in connection with skin nevi.

As expected, **skin carcinomas** were found in the older age groups (> 40). Less than one-tenth were observed in patients under the age of 40; the number gradually increased in the age groups above 40. No significant difference in sex was found, but there was a slight male preponderance with age. No differences in sex and age were observed in the remaining tumors, most of which consisted of benign epithelial cysts, epidermal and adnexal.

Previous Local Changes

A total of 39 patients had previous local changes in the same area as the present tumor. The sex distribution was equal.

A previous tumor was found in 30 of these cases; it was malignant in four cases. One of the latter patients has now presented with a benign papilloma in the same localization; for the other three treated earlier with diathermy or x-rays, the malignant tumor recurred. Of the 26 initially benign tumors, five recurred as malignant tumors. They had all been treated by excision (Table 1). They consisted of four epidermal tumors and one adnexal lid tumor.

Table 1   Recurrence of Tumors (Total: 30).

Primary Tumor	Therapy of Primary Tumor	Recurrence		Total
		"Recurred" as benign	"Recurred" as malignant	
Benign	Surgical therapy	20	5	
	Other therapy	1	–	26
Malignant	Surgical therapy	1	–	
	Other therapy	–	3	4
Total		22	8	30

The remaining nine cases of previous local changes were two cases of foreign body granuloma occurring after squint operations, two cases of organized hematoma after contusions and five cases with irrelevant changes.

Duration of Past History

The duration of the past history is shown in Diagram 2. We define duration as the period from the first observation of the tumor by the patient until diagnosis was made and treatment instituted. This information must, therefore, be taken with some reservation.

In regard to **congenital tumors**, the information of the clinical onset usually depends upon observations made by the parents. The congenital group in Diagram 2 is the only group which does not include malignant cases. The group is not composed entirely of children. This group of 15 patients was made up of six cases of nevi (one conjunctival nevus), one benign localized melanosis in the conjunctiva, three cysts (two dermoid cysts), and in the remaining five cases various epidermal tumors and one case of lymphangioma.

For the other groups in Diagram 2, it appears as if the past duration provides no specific, helpful clues for the clinician in assessing the individual case. No features could be demonstrated that allowed us to differentiate between a "benign" and a "malignant" history.

As is shown in Diagram 2, about 10% of the patients were unable to provide definite information regarding the history; this corresponds with clinical experience.

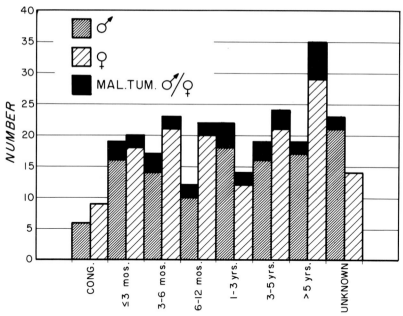

Diagram 2   Duration of Past History.
The diagram shows the duration of the past history for males and females in arbitrarily selected temporal groups.
The diagram also shows the number of malignant tumors within these groups

Symptoms

In general, the tumors in this series have been **symptomless**. Cosmetic inconvenience or the worry of bearing a serious lesion were the reasons for going to a physician.
Symptoms were found in only 37 patients, equally distributed according to sex. The complaints were mainly **conjunctival** (foreign-body sensation, itching and epiphora), and they were observed in all histological groups.
It is strange, however, that such symptoms were encountered in only 12 of 64 conjunctival tumors; all were localized on the palpebral conjunctiva. The majority of the palpebral tumors producing conjunctival symptoms were localized on the palpebral margin; they caused more inconvenience than the purely conjunctival tumors. In three cases **hemorrhage** was the reason for consultation; all lesions were basal cell carcinomas. **Visual disturbance** was found in only three patients; one of these patients was a child with unilateral amblyopia caused by a large lymphangioma from early childhood.

Signs

Localization of the Tumors (Table 2)

The skin around the lids, particularly the superciliary region and the skin area immediately outside the canthi, were the areas investigated; tumors in other areas of the facial skin were not considered unless they were found together with tumors localized in the above-mentioned areas relevant to this study.
The skin. The total number of tumors was 18. Nearly half of these were **dermoid cysts** (7). No dermoid cysts in this series were orbitopalpebral. Two skin tumors were **basal cell carcinomas**; the remaining were benign epidermal tumors and tumors of the dermal appendages.
The lid. The total number of lid tumors (218) was equally distributed on the upper and lower lids. A little more than half (125) were epidermal tumors, one-sixth (33) were adnexal, and

Table 2 Localization of Tumors

	Total Number	Number, Malignant
Skin outside eyelids	18	2
Skin of upper eyelid	117	6
Skin of lower eyelid	101	24
Palpebral conjunctiva	20	1
Bulbar conjunctiva	19	2
Caruncle	25	1
Total	300	36

one-ninth (24) were nevi. The remaining lesions were partly vascular and partly inflammatory, mainly molluscum contagiosum. Only one tumor showed a predilection for one of the lids: the number of **basal cell carcinomas** was significantly higher on the lower lid (24/101) than on the upper lid (6/117). This difference could possibly be explained by the greater exposure of the lower eyelid to actinic radiation. No significant difference in occurrence on the temporal and nasal part of the lid was found. The preferred location of basal cell carcinomas on the lower lid could not be correlated with any other tumor of the series, particularly not with papillomas. The finding emphasizes the fact that papillomas of the skin cannot be considered precancerous lesions, such as papillomas of the mucous membranes (e.g., in the colon and the urinary bladder).

Nevi appeared with equal frequency on upper and lower lids. However, the occurrence of nevi in women was twice as frequent as in men. This difference in the frequency of occurrence between the two sexes corresponds with other series of skin nevi (cf., sex and age distribution, p. 2).

The **vascular** and **inflammatory lesions** showed no difference, either in localization or in distribution between the sexes.

Conjunctiva. The 64 conjunctival tumors were subdivided according to their location: 20 were confined to the **palpebral** conjunctiva, 19 to the **bulbar** conjunctiva, and 25 to the **caruncle**. **Nevi** were frequent; they made up one-fifth of the palpebral and one-third of the bulbar and caruncular cases. In contrast to the cutaneous nevi (cf. p. 2), no difference between the sexes could be noted. **Epithelial cysts** followed the nevi in frequency. Two caruncular cases of **sebaceous adenoma** were found in males. Only four of the 64 conjunctival tumors were **malignant**, i.e., a squamous cell carcinoma at the limbus originating in a leukoplakia, a basal cell carcinoma of the caruncle, a cancerous melanosis of the palpebral conjunctiva, and a malignant melanoma of the bulbar conjunctiva.

Shape

The tumors were clinically divided into cystic, papillomatous, and nodular. No difference in sex or localization was found within these groups.

Cystic (Figs. 4, 5, 6, 15, 16, 17). Clinically, 84 tumors were classified as cystic. This impression was largely confirmed histopathologically, i.e., epidermal cysts, dermoid cysts, various cysts from the adnexal structures as well as some **nevi of the caruncle**, which are nearly always characterized by small epithelial inclusion cysts (as also found in some other conjunctival nevi).

The fact that three **basal cell carcinomas** were cystic may be more interesting (Fig. 12 A). Ectopic lacrimal gland tissue may often have a cystic appearance; it frequently clinically resembles a dermoid cyst (Fig. 32).

Papillomatous (Figs. 1, 2; Color Plate IV D). This shape applied to 128 tumors. The tumors were mainly **papillomas** of skin and conjunctiva. However, 15% of the total number were **basal cell carcinomas** (Fig. 9) and 15% were **nevi**.

Nodular (Figs. 7, 10, 13, 19; Color Plate IV G). A total of 85 tumors were classified as nodular. Histologically, no single type of tumor prevailed within this group. It is important to emphazise that small **nodular nevi** on the palpebral margin often resemble a fibroma (Fig. 19). Several **epidermal cysts** (Fig. 4) were included in this group of nodular tumors. Since they had been present for a long period of time, they had acquired a nodular noncystic appearance. Further, 11% of the nodular tumors were **basal cell carcinomas**.

Color

Distinction has been made between brown-pigmented, mainly melanocyte-containing tumors (Color Plate IV A), and blue or red, yellowish, and black tumors.

The **brown-pigmented** tumors were mainly **nevi**. Only two of the 16 brown-pigmented tumors found in males were not nevi (two pigmented papillomas); 12 of the 24 brown-pigmented tumors found in females were, however, not nevi, but various epidermal pigmented tumors (Color Plate I A, II A). Hypothetically, hormonal conditions may be responsible for this difference (cf. chloasmata in pregnant women).

We wish to emphasize that **nevi occurring before puberty in children** are often salmon-pink in color or even colorless. On the conjunctiva they may be completely transparent and present as small cysts (Fig. 21).

In regard to other colors, **blue or red** tumors were predominant. **Hemangiomas** or organized **hemorrhages** were found most frequently (Color Plate III D, F), but some skin **carcinomas** also acquire this color due to deep, proliferating vessels.

Epidermal cysts and a few **nevi**, as well as **sebaceous adenomas**, were mainly **yellowish** (Color Plate II F). **Keratoacanthoma** may also be yellowish (Color Plate I D). Old hemorrhages may be completely **black**.

Surface

The majority of the tumors (about 200) had a smooth uncharacteristic surface. The others could be subdivided into three categories according to their predominant clinical feature, i.e., scaling, ulcerating, and inflammatory appearance.

Scaling. By scaling, we mean that the skin above the tumor was covered by small keratinous scales, or small, loose, frayed skin flakes. A total of 44 tumors had this type of surface. They were mainly benign and malignant epithelial tumors. **Papillomas** constituted 30 (including two kerato-acanthomas) (Color Plate I D), while nine were **carcinomas** (three squamous cell carcinomas) (Fig. 10). It was unusual that three **epidermal cysts** had a scaling surface (Fig. 5). No conjunctival papillomas were described as having a scaling surface.

Ulcerating. A total of 20 tumors had an ulcerating surface. **Basal cell carcinomas** constituted 14 of these (Fig. 7; Color Plate II D). No ulcerating carcinomas were squamous cell carcinomas; this is a well-known fact (Fig. 10). The last six ulcerating cases were made up of four papillomas, a hemangioendotheliosarcoma (Color Plate III D) and an epidermal cyst.

Inflammatory appearance. A total of 14 lesions had an inflammatory appearance. Half of these were more or less **atypical chalazia**; the others were atypical xanthelasmata and molluscum contagiosum.

Mobility in Relation to the Substratum

Only 39 tumors adhered to the substratum; 40% (15) of these were **carcinomas** (11 basal cell carcinomas, three squamous cell carcinomas, and one sebaceous carcinoma). Eight **cystic lesions** (mainly dermoid cysts) adhered to the base; the remaining immobile tumors were **nevi** and **vascular** tumors.

Clinical Diagnosis

The tumors were clinically divided into nine groups, which experience has shown can be distinguished. These groups are shown in Table 3.

Table 3 Clinical Diagnosis

	Number	Percent
1. Papilloma	88	29
2. Carcinoma	27	9
3. Atheroma	28	10
4. Other cysts	46	15
5. Angiomas	12	4
6. Nevi/melanosis	40	13
7. Fibroma	10	3
8. Atypical chalazion	18	6
9. Miscellaneous	31	11
Total	300	100

A **papilloma** was a branching or lobulated tumor, pedunculated or with a broad base.
A **carcinoma,** in the clinical sense, was a firm, more or less nodular, often ulcerating tumor, which frequently adhered to the substratum.
Clinically, **atheromas** were cyst-like lesions with white or yellow contents.
Dermoid cysts were easily recognized clinically, and were included in the group of **cysts.**
By **angiomas,** the clinician meant rather soft, slightly elevated, red or bluish tumors of conjunctiva or skin.
Nevi were brown-pigmented, circumscribed, slightly elevated tumors of skin or conjunctiva; a **melanosis** was a diffusely brown-pigmented, non-elevated area.
A **fibroma** was a solid, slightly elevated, apparently unpigmented tumor, partly adhering to the substratum; it was often localized on the margin of the lid.
An **atypical chalazion** was a chalazion-like nodule, localized on the inside of the lids. The patient was frequently referred because the practicing ophthalmologist suspected a malignant tumor.
A lesion which could not easily be placed in one of the above groups was placed in the **miscellaneous** group.
Correlation between the clinical and histopathological diagnoses will be given below (Table 4).

Table 4 Comparison of Clinical and Histopathological Diagnoses

Clinical Diagnosis	Main Histopathological Groups									
	Benign epiderm.	Malign. epiderm.	Benign adnex.	Malign. adnex.	Neuro-genous	Vascu-lar	Mesoder-mal	Inflam.	Miscel.	Total
1. Papilloma	68	6	–	–	12	–	–	2	–	88
2. Carcinoma	4	21	–	–	–	1	–	1	–	27
3. Atheroma	18	2	5	–	–	1	–	2	–	28
4. Other cysts	33	2	–	–	–	4	–	2	5	46
5. Angiomas	5	–	–	–	2	5	–	–	–	12
6. Nevi/melanosis	5	–	3	–	31	–	–	1	–	40
7. Fibroma	–	1	–	–	6	–	3	–	–	10
8. Atyp. chalaz.	1	2	1	–	2	–	–	12	–	18
9. Miscellaneous	–	–	–	–	–	–	–	–	31	31
Total										300

In the total material (excluding the miscellaneous group), a discrepancy between the clinical and histopathological diagnoses was found in 33% of cases (89/269). Five percent of the benign groups (groups 1, 3–8) proved to be malignant tumors clinically evaluated as benign. This finding stresses the importance of a histopathological examination of **all** tissue removed. In addition, five of the malignant tumors in this series were recurrences of apparently benign tumors, which were previously removed unradically and without histopathological examination. On the other hand, 22% of the tumors clinically diagnosed as carcinomas proved to be benign.

The clinical evaluations in the nine diagnostic groups are discussed briefly below in relation to histopathological verification.

Papilloma

Clinical evaluation: 88 cases.
Correct diagnosis: 68 cases (six conjunctival [Fig. 3]).
Incorrect diagnosis: 20 cases (22%). These comprised:
  6 carcinomas (four basal cell, one squamous cell and one mixed [= basosquamous] [Fig. 9 A]);
12 neurogenous tumors (one apigmented nevus [Color Plate IV D], 10 pigmented, and one
    neurinoma);
  2 atypical chalazia (Color Plate IV G).

Carcinoma

Clinical evaluation: 27 cases.
Correct diagnosis: 21 cases (basal cell and squamous cell carcinomas).
Incorrect diagnosis: 6 cases (four papillomas, one hemangioendotheliosarcoma [Color Plate III D], and one hypertrophic chalazion).

Atheroma

Clinical evaluation: 28 cases.
Correct diagnosis: 16 cases.
Incorrect diagnosis: 12 cases (five benign adnexal tumors [Fig. 12 B], two basal cell carcinomas [non-ulcerating], one hemangioma, and two chalazia; two papillomas are included in Table 4, grouped with benign epidermal tumors).

Other Cysts

Clinical evaluation: 46 cases.
Correct diagnosis: 33 cases.
Incorrect diagnosis: 13 cases (30%) (two basal cell carcinomas, two lymphangiomas [Fig. 28], two hemangiomas, two lymphomas, and two cases of ectopic lacrimal gland tissue [Fig. 32]; the remaining three were benign epithelial tumors.

Angioma

Clinical evaluation: 12 cases.
Correct diagnosis: 5 cases.
Incorrect diagnosis: 7 cases.
The high percentage of error was due possibly to hemorrhages in various cystic tumors and heavy pigmentation in two nevi.

Nevus (Color Plate IV A, D)

Clinical evaluation: 40 cases.
Correct diagnosis: 31 cases.
Incorrect diagnosis: 9 cases (five papillomas, three adnexal tumors and one foreign body granuloma). One of the "nevi" turned out to be a malignant conjunctival melanoma.

Fibroma

Clinical evaluation: 10 cases.
Correct diagnosis: 3 cases.
Incorrect diagnosis: 7 cases (six unpigmented intradermal nevi, one carcinoma [Fig. 9 B]). The unpigmented intradermal nevus localized on the palpebral margin clinically presents as a firm fibrous nodule (Fig. 19).

Atypical Chalazion (Color Plate IV G)

Clinical evaluation: 18 cases.
Correct diagnosis: 12 cases.
Incorrect diagnosis: 6 cases (one papilloma, one hypertrophic sebaceous gland, two carcinomas, and two nevi). A localized nodular lesion with the appearance of a chalazion, but somewhat firmer, was most often referred because the ophthalmologist suspected a malignant neoplasm or a lesion other than a chalazion. The two cases of carcinoma justified the referral of the remaining 16 non-malignant cases.

Miscellaneous

Clinical evaluations: 31 cases.
Correct diagnosis: 9 cases.
Incorrect diagnosis: 22 cases.
This group was composed of the less frequent clinical diagnoses (molluscum contagiosum, "granuloma", lymphoma, lipoma).

The diagnoses were correct in cases of **molluscum contagiosum** and **granulomas**; here the history is often of great importance. The reason for the high percentage of error in this group was because these special tumors do not have a characteristic clinical appearance. Some cases, e.g., clinically diagnosed lymphoma, were simple epidermal cysts and some pterygia; a few tumors which clinically appeared to be granulomas proved to be intradermal nevi and epidermal cysts. Only one malignant tumor in this group (a reticulosarcoma [Fig. 33]) was correctly diagnosed clinically.

Histopathology

The main histopathological groups are shown in Table 5. A total of 319 tumors were found in the 300 patients; 19 patients had two tumors removed, all benign. In 13 patients, the two tumors were similar but in different locations, i.e., upper and/or lower eyelid, skin of eyelid, and/or palpebral conjunctiva. The remaining six cases were nevi combined with different benign epithelial and adnexal tumors.

Table 5 Survey of Histopathological Groups

Groups	Number			Percent
	M	F	Total	
Benign epidermal tumors	64	73	137	44
Malignant epidermal tumors	19	15	34	10
Benign adnexal tumors	9	10	19	6
Malignant adnexal tumors	2	–	2	1
Neurogenous tumors	21	33	54	17
Vascular tumors	4	8	12	3
Mesodermal soft tissue tumors	3	2	5	2
Inflammations	15	19	34	11
Choristomas (dermoid cysts)	3	8	11	3
Miscellaneous	4	7	11	3
Total	144	175	319	100

The correlation between the clinical diagnosis and the main histopathological groups is shown in Table 4 (p. 7). This table shows the main clinical groups distributed between the main histopathological groups; it should be read from left to right.

In terms of histopathology (Table 5), the largest subgroup comprises the **benign epidermal tumors**; they account for nearly half (44%) of the total series. This subgroup is further subdivided (Table 6) according to histological criteria. Almost two thirds of the benign epidermal tumors were **papillomas**, mainly **keratotic papillomas** (= squamous cell papillomas, 45%) (Fig. 1). Next in frequency came **epidermal cysts** (25 per cent) (Figs. 4, 5). Separating these from the so-called

Table 6 Benign Epidermal Tumors

Diagnoses	Number			Percent
	M	F	Total	
Keratotic papilloma (squamous cell p.)	30	32	62	45
Basal cell papilloma (seborrheic keratosis)	4	7	11	8
Conjunctival papilloma	5	5	10	8
Epidermal cyst	17	17	34	25
Keratoacanthoma	–	1	1	1
Pilomatrixoma (Calc. ep. of Malherbe)	1	–	1	
Various simple cysts	7	11	18	13
Total	64	73	137	100

sebaceous cysts originating in dilated sebaceous ducts is often impossible, and has therefore not been undertaken in the present work.

Basal cell papilloma (= seborrheic keratosis) (Fig. 2) and **conjunctival papilloma** (Fig. 3) each constituted 8%.

Keratoacanthoma (Color Plate I D–F) and **pilomatrixoma** (= benign calcifying epithelioma of Malherbe) (Color Plate I G, H) were each encountered only once. The latter tumor is seldom diagnosed clinically.

Malignant epidermal tumors (Table 5) comprised 10% of the total series. About four-fifths were basal cell carcinomas; the rest, squamous cell carcinomas. **Basal cell carcinoma** (Figs. 7, 8; Color Plate II D–E) possesses the ability of invasive growth and deep ulceration (rodent ulcer) but is considered relatively benign because of the slow progress and lack of metastases. Three-quarters of basal cell carcinomas of the series had been present for at least three years; only one in four had a history of less than one year. In regard to morphology, two-thirds of the cases appeared as nodular tumors with ulceration; one-third were papillomatous or in other ways atypical.

Squamous cell carcinoma (Fig. 10) is a malignant skin tumor with metastasizing potentiality and usually a shorter history than that of the basal cell carcinoma. Four of the seven squamous cell carcinomas had been present for less than one year. They appeared as papillomatous tumors without ulceration. In a few cases, diathermy had been performed, sometimes repeatedly, since the tumors were considered to be simple papillomas. Only one case was localized in the conjunctiva (Fig. 11). We have no evidence that the carcinomas originated in actinic keratosis. The **benign adnexal tumors** (Table 5) constituted 6% of the total number. They were mainly sebaceous adenomas or hyperplasia of sebaceous glands (Figs. 12, 13, 14; Color Plate II F, G, H) but a few suderiferous cysts (Moll cysts) (Figs. 15, 16) and syringocystadenomas appeared (Fig. 17).

The series contained only two **malignant adnexal tumors**, both arising from meibomian glands (Color Plate III A, B, C). These tumors tend to recur when not properly treated; metastases may even be seen.

The distribution of the **neurogenous tumors** is specified in Table 7. These tumors constituted 17% (see Table 5) (p. 10). **Nevi** were by far the most frequent type of tumor. Considering the total number of nevi in all localizations, the interesting sex and age difference has already been emphasized (p. 2).

Table 7   Neurogenous Tumors and Their Localization

		M	F		Total number
Nevi	Skin	8	23	31	
	Conjunctiva	7	3	10	50
	Caruncle	5	4	9	
Malignant pigmented tumors		–	2		2
Schwannoma		1	1		2
Total		21	33		54

The majority of the cutaneous nevi were intradermal (75%) (Figs. 19, 20; Color Plate IV A, B, C). About one-third (15) of the cutaneous, conjunctival, and caruncular nevi belonged to the junctional and compound types (Figs. 18, 21, 22, 23, 24; Color Plate IV D, E, F). Only three of these cases were patients over the age of 30.

Only two malignant pigmented tumors were encountered, i.e., a case of precancerous, perhaps **cancerous, melanosis**, and a case of a solid conjunctival **malignant melanoma**. Clinically, the diagnosis was a benign melanosis and a nevus respectively.

One of the cases of **Schwannoma** was clinically diagnosed as a papilloma; the other was recognized in a previously diagnosed Recklinghausen's disease.

The **vascular tumors** (see Table 5) (3%) were mainly various **hemangiomas** (Figs. 25, 27; Color Plate III, F, G, H), including two sclerosing hemangiomas (Fig. 26) and one malignant **hemangio-endothelioma** (Color Plate III D, E). We considered two **lymphangiomas** (Fig. 28) in this group. No prevailing age groups could be established within this group of tumors.

There were surprisingly few **mesodermal soft tissue tumors** (2%) compared with the clinical diagnosis (see Table 3: fibroma) (p. 7). This is probably because nevi are very often diagnosed by the clinician as fibromas (see Table 4) (p. 7). Histopathologically, this group was composed of scar tissue, fibromas, and a myxoma (Fig. 29).

The **inflammatory tumors** (11%) were atypical **chalazia** in more than half the cases (Color Plate IV G, H). Recurrences of previously removed chalazia were found particularly in this group (Fig. 30 C, D). Of the total number, one in four were **foreign body granulomas** (some after squint operations) and connective tissue with simple inflammation. Five cases of **molluscum contagiosum** concurred with the clinical diagnosis. We included three cases of benign **lymphoma** (Fig. 30 A, B) in this group; all were elderly patients. All of the cases had been misinterpreted by the clinician before surgery.

Choristomas constituted 3%. These were all **dermoid cysts** usually found in children in the lateral part of the supercilium, but may be found anywhere around the eye. They can be mistaken for other benign lesions (Fig. 32).

In the **miscellaneous** group (3%), two cases of ectopic lacrimal gland tissue were found (Fig. 32). Clinically, the correct diagnosis was proposed in one case, while the other was diagnosed as a dermoid cyst (cf. Figs. 31, 32). One of two cases of xanthelasma was regarded as an atheroma. Two simple cysts located in the caruncle were regarded as a papilloma and a dermoid cyst respectively; one case of reticulosarcoma (Fig. 33) was diagnosed clinically as a sarcoma of the dermis. The remaining tumors were various clinically uncharacteristic mesodermal lesions, mainly scar tissue.

Summarizing for the whole series, the clinical and histopathological diagnoses concurred in 66% (199/300) of cases.

The corrections of the clinical evaluations were not influenced by sex or age.

Treatment

All tumors which were clearly benign clinically were totally excised. Epithelial tumors where the slightest clinical suspicion of malignancy was present were treated as follows:

1. Open marginal biopsy (Fig. 34).
2. Postoperative irradiation with x-rays (50–60 KV) if malignant, about 4500 R/10 days.

It is important that the marginal biopsy is deep, including viable tumor tissue (not possibly necrotic areas) as well as the tumor margin and the adjacent normal skin. Suturing is not necessary when only a 2-mm-thick slice is removed.
We recommend this procedure because:

a) Radical surgical excision is often difficult due to the localization of the tumor near the lid margin or the lacrimal ductules; this eventually causes ectropion, entropion and/or stenosis of lacrimal ductules. A radical procedure often requires major plastic surgery.
b) It is extremely important that the radiotherapist be informed of the exact size and appearance of the lesion so that he can correctly adjust the field and the radiation dose. Frequently, in an excision, the scar is considerably larger than the original lesion. This often results in the use of a larger radiation field than necessary, and therefore a greater tendency toward radiation-induced scar formation.
c) It is important that the vessels nourishing the lesion are preserved, since the optimal effect of radiation is dependent upon the oxygen supply which is guaranteed by an intact connective tissue stroma. Nourishing vessels will not be intact if radiation is applied to a scar after an excision.
d) The procedure produces a cosmetically satisfactory result. The biopsy can always be performed under local anesthesia and is not as drastic as major surgery might be. Surgical treatment, when properly carried out, can have equally good results. Radical excision (at least 5 mm of healthy tissue around and beneath a basal cell carcinoma and 10 mm around a squamous cell carcinoma), however, necessitates plastic reconstruction of the lids; not all ophthalmologists are prepared for this.

In the event of pigmented lesions we recommend a somewhat different procedure, because traumatization is undesirable here. The danger is malignant transformation of a benign lesion or increased metastatic tendency in a malignant one.

a) In the event of a nevus on the lid or conjunctiva, it is recommended that total excision be attempted. If the histopathological examination reveals a malignant melanoma, major plastic surgery must be performed subsequently.
b) In the event of conjunctival melanosis, an attempt should be made to excise a more limited part, preferably an elevated area with a malignant appearance. If the melanosis proves to be malignant, orbital exenteration is necessary. If it proves to be precancerous, no definite policy can be recommended; observation and surgery may be a possibility.

Follow-Up

The follow-up included all malignant cases, precancerous lesions, and some other cases which may transform into a malignant lesion, although the possibility is slight (cf. Table 5) (p. 10).

1. The number of **basal cell carcinomas** was 25. The observation period ranged from six to eight years. Two patients died. One patient died from a metastasizing breast carcinoma one year after treatment of the lid tumor; the other, from a carcinoma of the stomach five years later.

The remaining 23 patients were all alive and well. A reticulosarcoma of the stomach had been removed surgically in one patient.

There was only one local recurrence of an irradiated basal cell carcinoma, which occurred after three years. It was treated by plastic surgery.

2. The **squamous cell carcinomas** (seven patients) had no local or general recurrence. Four of the patients, however, died one to five years after treatment (two died of bronchopneumonia, one of carcinoma of the colon, and one of a prostatic carcinoma).

3. One **meibomian carcinoma** recurred eight months after treatment. This patient had metastases in the cervical glands, but underwent plastic surgery and is still alive seven years later. The other patient with a meibomian carcinoma had no recurrence of the tumor, but died six years after treatment from a metastasizing colon carcinoma.

Without investigating the statistics, it is remarkable that seven of 32 patients had a malignant neoplasm elsewhere, although not at the same time as the malignant lid tumor. This, however, corresponds with a large series of malignant neoplasms where the occurrence of multiple cancer is more frequent than might be accounted for by pure chance.

4. Two patients had **malignant pigmented tumors.** In one, a circumscribed malignant melanoma of the conjunctiva was excised broadly; no further therapy was applied. This patient is alive five years after excision, without local or general recurrence. The other had a precancerous conjunctival melanosis. Repeated biopsies showed increasing malignancy leading to exenteration of the orbit two years after the first biopsy. The patient died with cerebral and lymph node metastases three years later; i.e., five years after the first biopsy.

5. One of the three cases of **lymphoma** recurred as a lymphosarcoma in the orbit two years later. The patient was treated with betatron and mobaltron radiation but died of generalized lymphosarcoma five years after the initial lesion. The remaining two patients had no recurrence.

6. The patient with **reticulosarcoma** (cf., Fig. 33) of the lower lid had bilateral choroidal involvement after five years and died from cerebral reticulosarcoma six years after radiation therapy for the primary tumor.

7. All the **vascular** tumors were followed up. No recurrence or death occurred in this group. All irradiated cases showed a good functional and cosmetic result (Fig. 35).

Atlas

Color Plate I

A. (Rec. no. 172, Lab. no. 464/68) **Pigmented keratotic papilloma.**
   52-year-old female with a tumor for 8 to 10 years, rapidly growing in the last 3 months. Local irritation. Tumor also on margin of lid and a few millimeters on the palpebral side. Lobulated, with a few hairs on the surface. Clinically designated as pigmented papilloma.

B. Survey of section showing the papillomatous surface and the sharp stromal border (x 25).

C. The pigmented basal cells along the stromal border can be seen, giving the tumor clinically its pigmented appearance (x 100).

D. (Rec. no. 14, Lab. no. 500/68) **Keratoacanthoma.**
   57-year-old female with a pea-sized, scaling, rapidly growing tumor for 3 months on margin of lower lid. Adherent to the base.

E. The survey shows the cup-shaped formation with the keratin-filled cup and the cup-forming epithelial masses (x 25).

F. The acanthotic epithelial part. The keratin lamellas are in the upper right corner (x 100).

G. (Rec. no. 81, Lab. no. 34/66) **Pilomatrixoma (calcifying epithelioma of Malherbe).**
   11-year-old boy with a tumor in left superciliary region for 2 months. One month prior to operation, he received a blow toward the supercilium; the tumor subsequently became red.

H. Section showing the shadow cells *(arrow)* and a calcification *(double arrow)*. Viable epithelial cells are seen in the upper right corner (x 100).

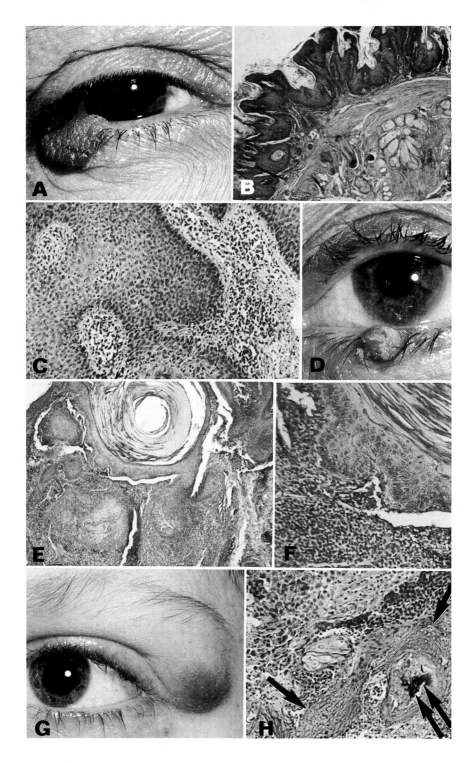

Color Plate I

Color Plate II

A. (Rec. no. 3, Lab. no. 458/68 + 764/68) **Trichoepithelioma.**
52-year-old man with a firm tumor on lower eyelid for 1 year. Adherent to the base. Foreign-body sensation.

B. Survey of tumor showing epithelial masses and horn cysts (x 25).

C. A horn cyst (pilar cyst) with a rudimentary hair centrally (x 100).

D. (Rec. no. 116, Lab. no. 179/68) **Advanced basal cell carcinoma.**
88-year-old man with a slowly expanding ulceration at inner canthus. No involvement of nose, nasolacrimal duct, or bulbus. The whole lower lid infiltrated by tumor tissue.

E. Section showing the ulcerated surface covered with blood, and the infiltrating epithelial strands (x 25). See also Fig. 8.

F. (Rec. no. 166, Lab. no. 142/66) **Sebaceous adenoma of the caruncle.**
42-year-old man with slowly growing white spot at inner angle for some months.

G. The tumor is composed of solid islands of closely packed sebaceous cells (x 25).

H. The cells have light, slightly granulated cytoplasm and a prominent nucleus (x 250).

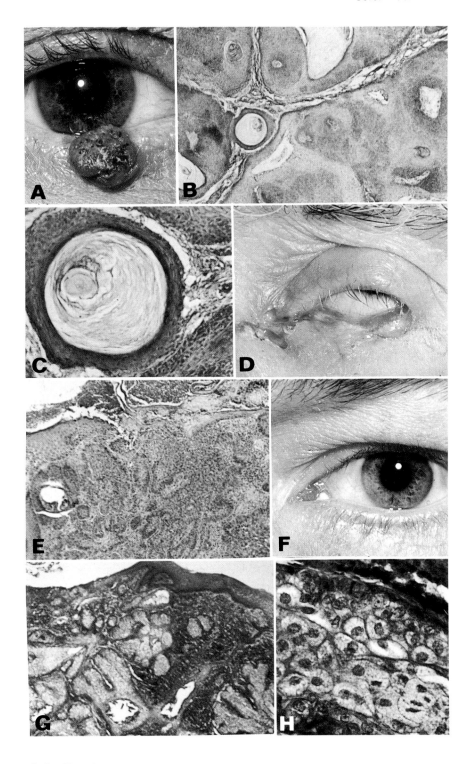

Color Plate II

Color Plate III

A. (Rec. no. 124, Lab. no. 1/66) **Sebaceous adenoma with dedifferentiation.**
56-year-old man with a slowly growing yellow tumor for 1 year on the margin of the left upper lid. The tumor was solid.

B. Closely packed lobular formations of differentiated sebaceous cells. In the left side, dedifferentiated masses are present *(arrow)* (x 25).

C. Higher magnification of sebaceous cells and more dedifferentiated strands (x 250).

D. (Rec. no. 62, Lab. no. 649/68) **Hemangioendotheliosarcoma.**
58-year-old woman; tumor present for 3 months. Electrocoagulated 20 months after origin. Recurrence after three weeks. Rapid growth. Local irritation. Clinically thought to be a keratotic papilloma or a squamous carcinoma.

E. The lesion is composed of vascular spaces lined with atypical endothelial cells. Several mitoses are seen *(arrows)* (x 250).

F. (Rec. no. 257, Lab. no. 49/66) **Arteriovenous hemangioma.**
58-year-old woman with palpebral cyst of constant size for 4 to 5 years. It was soft with a small keratosis at lower margin.

G. The tumor is composed of thin-walled and thicker-walled vascular spaces, mostly filled with erythrocytes (x 25).

H. Confluent vascular spaces in higher magnification showing the thick vascular walls (x 250).

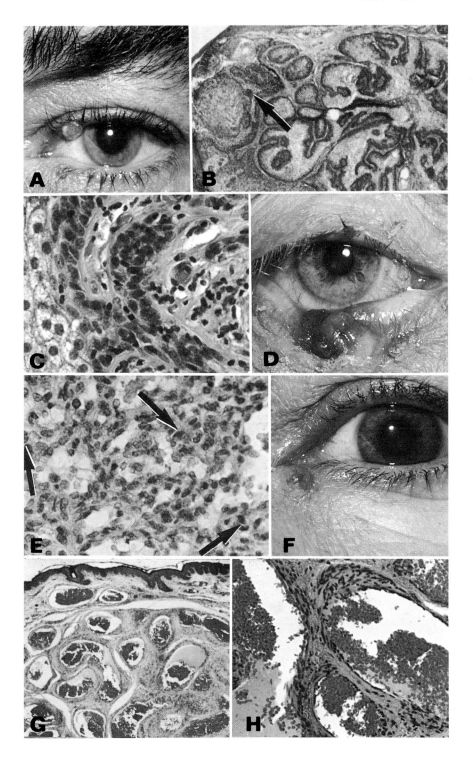

Color Plate III

Color Plate IV

A. (Rec. no. 177, Lab. no. 447/68) **Intradermal nevus of skin.**
   21-year-old woman with a pigmented lesion from the age of 11, which grew slowly until the patient was 18 years of age.

B. The nevoid structures, partly pigmented, are lying in the stroma (x 25).

C. Note the free stromal zone between the basal cells of the epithelium and the islands of nevus cells (x 100). See also Fig. 19 B.

D. (Rec. no. 238, Lab. no. 540/65) **Complex nevus of caruncle.**
   61-year-old woman. The tumor had been growing on the right caruncle for a few years. Clinically, it had the appearance of a papilloma.

E. In addition to the nevoid islands *(left)*, the tumor is composed of deeper-lying strands of tissue with neuroid structure *(arrow)* (x 25).

F. The neuroid structure resembling Meissner tactile corpuscles (x 250).

G. (Rec. no. 92, Lab. no. 647/67) **Atypical chalazion.**
   45-year-old man with a firm, pale tumor on left lower lid present for a few years. No growth. Clinically appearing as an unpigmented nevus (see Fig. 19 A).

H. The fibrous chalazion-like structure is seen (cf. Fig. 36 D) (x 25).

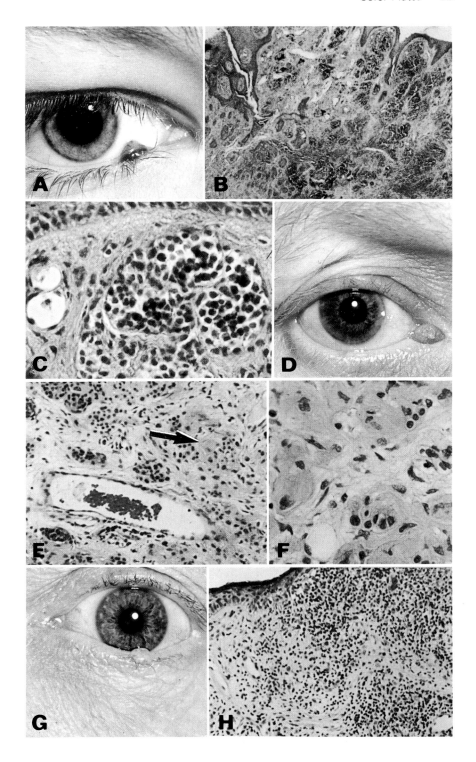

Color Plate IV

Benign Epidermal Tumors

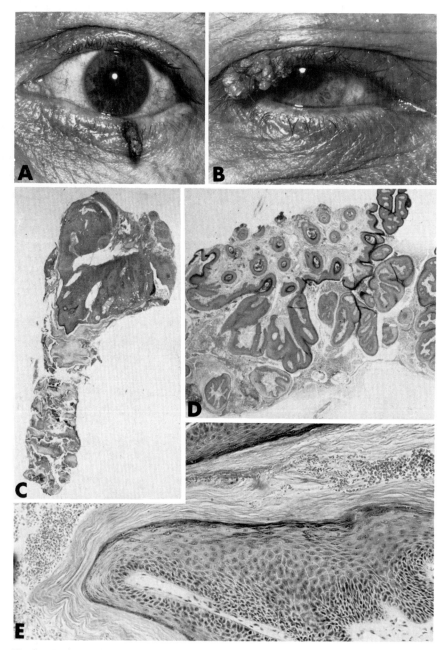

Fig. 1

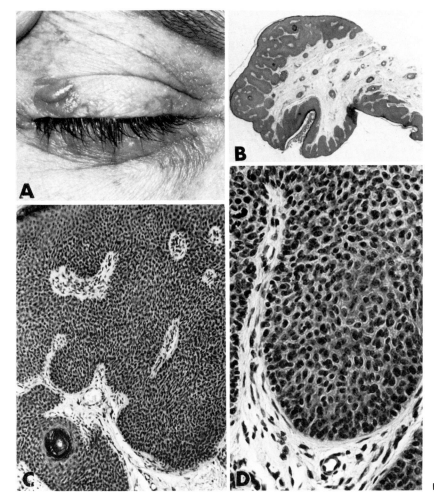

Fig. 2

Fig. 1. Keratotic papilloma.

A. (Rec. no. 117, Lab. no. 725/66).
Cutaneous horn (variety of the keratotic papilloma). 48-year-old man with cutaneous horn, recurring 2 years after simple removal.

B. (Rec. no. 02, Lab. no. 159/67).
55-year-old man with verruciform lesion for 4 to 5 years. Rapid growth for the last 3 to 4 months.

C. and D. Survey of the two keratotic lesions (x 10).

E. The lesions are composed of a connective tissue core covered with a hyperplastic stratified squamous epithelium producing abundant keratin. The sharp border against the stroma is seen (x 100).

Fig. 2. Basal cell papilloma (Seborrheic keratosis, verruca senilis).

A. (Rec. no. 281, Lab. no. 470/67).
63-year-old woman with brown verruca plana-like lesion for 10 years. It was adherent to the skin, but freely movable against the base.

B. Survey of the lesion showing the smooth surface and the broad connective tissue core (x 10).

C. Solid epithelial masses around tangentially-cut connective tissue processes; a small keratotic cyst in the left corner (x 100).

D. The border against the stroma is sharp. The cells are uniform and without mitoses (x 275).

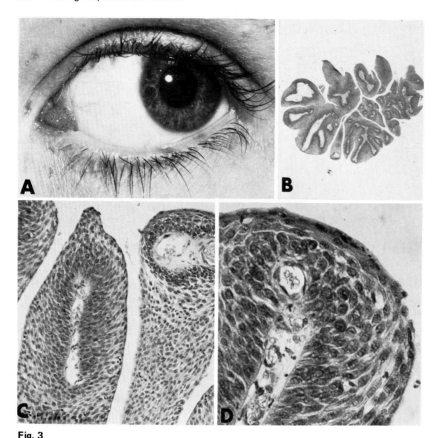

Fig. 3

Fig. 3. Papilloma of the caruncle.

A. (Rec. no. 151, Lab. no. 165/67).
17-year-old woman had a slowly-growing lobulated tumor for 2 to 3 months.

B. Survey of the tumor showing the papillomatous surface (x 10).

C. The connective tissue core is covered by hyperplastic conjunctival epithelium (x 100).

D. In high magnification, parakeratosis of superficial cells may be seen (x 275). A conjunctival papilloma outside the caruncle has basi-
cally the same clinical and histopathological
appearance.

Fig. 4. Epidermal cyst. ▶

A. (Rec. no. 85, Lab. no. 561/68).
72-year-old man with a slowly-growing yellow
palpebral tumor for several years.

B. (Rec. no. 230, Lab. no. 144/66).
64-year-old woman with a slowly-growing tumor from early childhood. It was soft and freely movable against the base.

C. Survey of the typical cyst. The epithelial lining
and the lumen filled with keratin lamellas are
characteristic (x 25).

D. Higher magnification of the wall showing the
stratified squamous epithelium and the keratin
lamellas. No adnexal structures (hairs or sebaceous glands) are to be found in the wall (x 100).

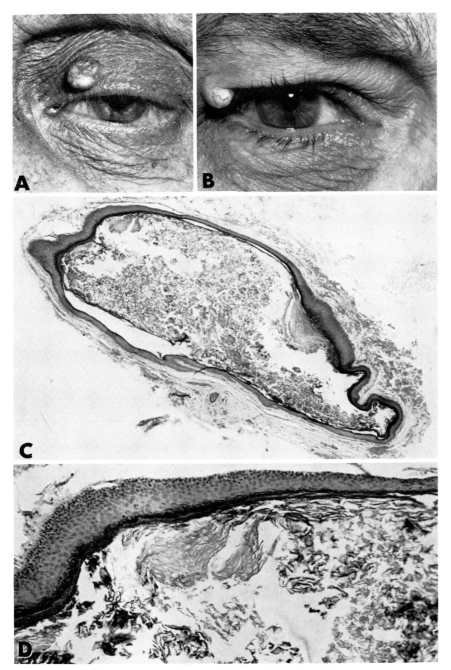

Fig. 4

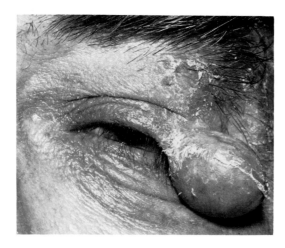

Fig. 5. Monstrous epidermal cyst.

(Rec. no. 239, Lab. no. 269/68).
49-year-old man with tumor for 7 to 8
years. It was soft and movable against
the base. Clinical diagnosis: lipoma. The
microscopical structure is similar to
Figure 4 C and D.

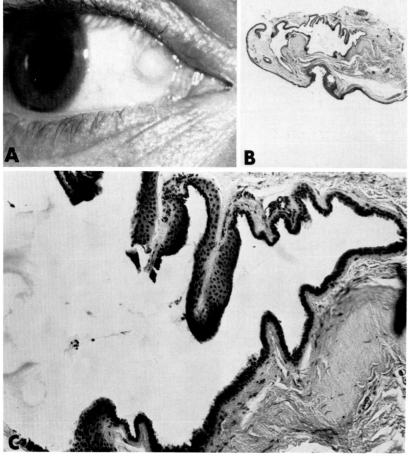

Fig. 6. Conjunctival cy

A. (Rec. no. 106, Lab
   no. 68/66).
   27-year-old woman
   had this cyst in the
   conjunctiva for 6
   months.

B. Survey of the part
   compressed cyst (x

C. The cyst wall is
   composed of an
   epithelium with
   varying layers of
   cells, from a few to
   several. No goblet
   cells are observed. T
   lumen is empty, bu
   probably contained
   serous fluid in vivo
   (x 100).

Malignant Epidermal Tumors

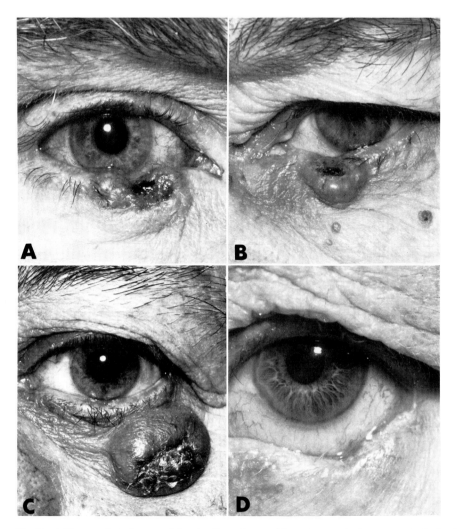

Fig. 7. Different clinical types of basal cell carcinoma. The microscopical structure is similar for all the lesions and is reproduced in Figure 8.

A. (Rec. no. 28, Lab. no. 650/66).
   50-year-old man with rapidly-growing ulcerating tumor for 6 months. Growth through lid and involvement of conjunctiva. Clinical diagnosis: basal cell carcinoma.

B. (Rec. no. 89, Lab. no. 743/66).
   82-year-old woman. Lid tumor for some months, rapidly growing. Adherent to skin, ulcerated with crust. Clinical diagnosis: "malignant tumor".

C. (Rec. no. 229, Lab. no. 207/67).
   57-year-old man with a slowly-growing ulcerating lesion for 10 years. No symptoms at any time. Partially adherent to skin, but not to underlying integument. Clinical diagnosis: "malignant tumor".

D. (Rec. no. 21, Lab. no. 119/66).
   76-year-old man with slowly growing, yellowish, firm lesion for 3 years; skin and conjunctiva involved. Clinically suspected to be a carcinoma. This form manifesting itself as a defect in the lid margin is quite typical of a basal cell carcinoma.

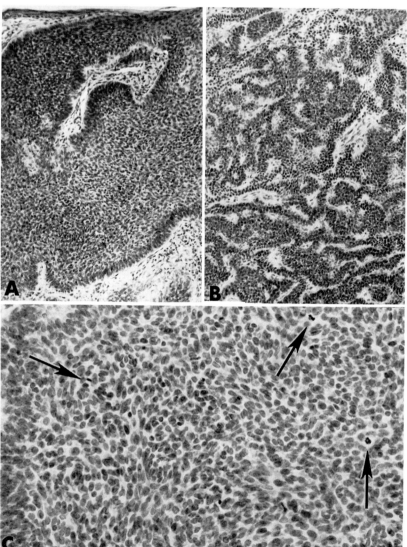

Fig. 8. Morphological patterns of basal cell circinoma.

A. (Rec. no. 21, Lab. no. 119/60).
The typical solid tissue from surface epithelium; the dermis is invaded. The cells are fairly uniform. In the periphery, palisading cells (x 100).

B. Various tissue patterns are often seen such as in this plexiform, alveolar, or adenoid type. The various patterns may be seen in the same tumor, such as is the case here (x 100).

C. At high magnification, several mitoses are often found (*arrows*). Pleomorphism is slight (x 275).

Fig. 9. Clinically atypical basal cell carcinomas. ▶

A. (Rec. no. 47, Lab. no. 778/65).
65-year-old man. Slowly-growing tumor of the caruncle region for 4 to 5 years. Adherent to skin of superior lid and to conjunctiva of inferior fornix. Clinical diagnosis: papilloma.

B. (Rec. no. 12, Lab. no. 90/66).
65-year-old man. Slowly-growing flat tumor without ulceration for several years. Adherent to skin. Clinical diagnosis: leukoplakia or fibroma.

C. (Rec. no. 47, Lab. no. 778/65).
Survey of the pedunculated invasive tumor of the caruncle (x 10).

D. (Rec. no. 12, Lab. no. 90/66).
Survey of the flat tumor showing no ulceration, but solid invasive tumor tissue.

E. The common morphological picture of the two lesions, showing the typical solid basal cell carcinoma with peripheral palisading of cells. A typical mitosis is seen (*arrow*) (x 275).

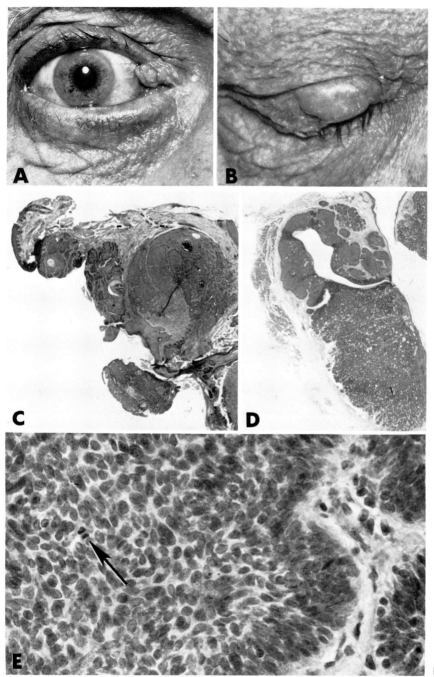

Fig. 9

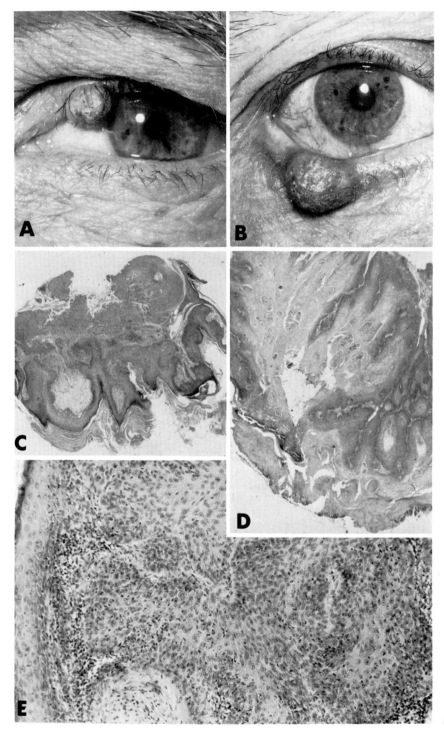

Fig. 10

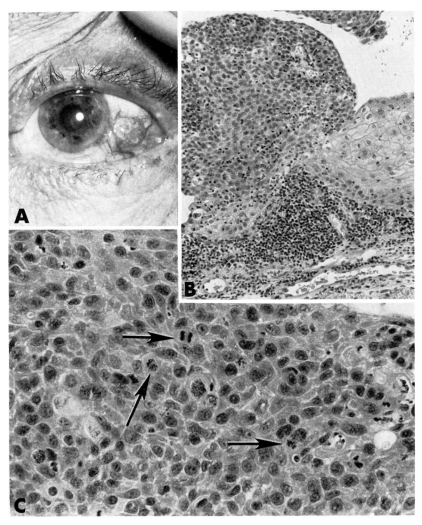

Fig. 11. Squamous cell carcinoma of conjunctiva.

A. (Rec. no. 196, Lab. no. 761/66). 70-year-old man with tumor for three weeks, slowly-growing, not adherent; large vessels toward tumor.

B. Survey of tumor showing a somewhat pedunculated structure. Heavy lymphocyte infiltration at the base. To the right, fairly normal epithelium (x 25).

C. The tumor is somewhat pleomorphic. Several mitoses are seen *(arrows)* (x 275).

◀ Fig. 10. Squamous cell carcinoma.

A. (Rec no. 136, Lab. no. 278/66). 64-year-old man with a slowly-growing nodular tumor for 4 to 5 years. Clinical diagnosis: verruca.

B. (Rec. no. 104, Lab. no. 23/68). 66-year-old man. Solid bluish tumor, rapidly growing for a few months, producing ectropion. Adherent to underlying skin but no involvement of the conjunctiva. No ulceration but scaling on top. Clinical diagnosis: "carcinoma".

C. and D. Survey of the tumors. The surface is covered with keratin. Solid tissue strands are invading the stroma *(above)* (x 10).

E. The typical squamous cell carcinoma is composed of oval and spindle cells in irregular masses which invade the dermis. Ulceration of the epithelium is not usually seen. Varying grades of differentiation are found. In the most differentiated types, horn pearls and intercellular bridges are seen. In the present case, no pearls were found (Broders' grade III) (x 100).

Benign Adnexal Tumors

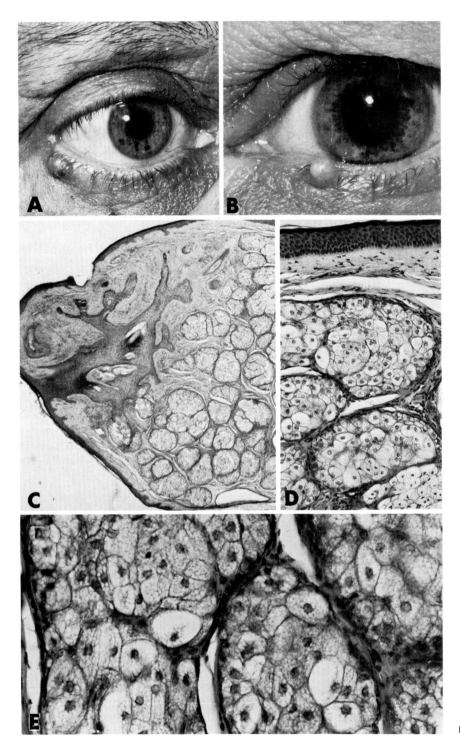

Fig. 12

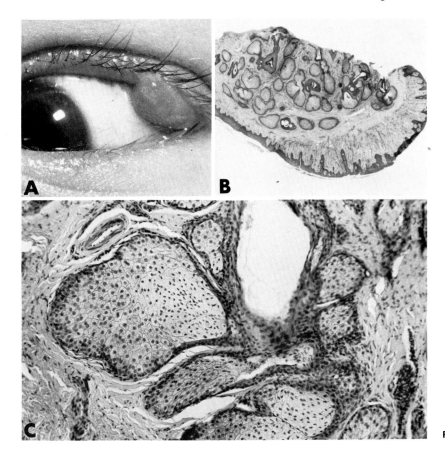

Fig. 13

◄ **Fig. 12. Basal cell carcinoma and sebaceous adenoma. Comparison to show the difficulty often met in clinical differentiation.**

A. (Rec. no. 27, Lab. no. 482/66).
   52-year-old woman with a slowly-growing, yellow-white, firm, but apparently cystic, tumor; delicate scales on the surface for a few years. Histological diagnosis: basal cell carcinoma. Microscopical structure: see Figure 8.

B. (Rec. no. 128, Lab. no. 76/66).
   46-year-old woman. A yellow-white, firm tumor without scales was present for several years on the lower lid margin.

C, D and E.
   The sebaceous adenoma consists of clusters of well-defined, clear, somewhat pleomorphic cells with a central round nucleus. In high magnification (E), the granulated cytoplasm is seen (x 10, x 100, x 275).

▲
Fig. 13. Hyperplasia of meibomian glands.

A. (Rec. no. 94, Lab. no. 79/66).
   One-year-old girl with congenital, reddish tumor growing for some weeks. Clinically, suspicion of hemangioma.

B. The hyperplastic glands are divided by solid strands of connective tissue, which differentiates the hyperplasia from an adenoma (cf. Fig. 14).

C. The glands are composed of small, uniform, light cells with small, central nuclei (x 100).

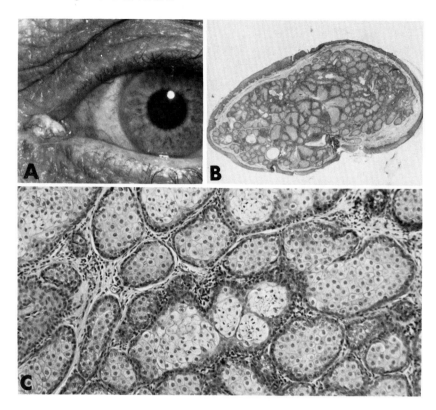

Fig. 14

Fig. 14. Sebaceous adenoma of the caruncle.

A. (Rec. no. 42, Lab. no. 473/65).
51-year-old man with yellow, lobulated, solid tumor of unknown duration. Clinical diagnosis: "caruncle tumor".

B. Survey of the excised tumor showing the epithelium-covered surface (x 10).

C. The tumor is composed of lobules of closely packed cells with light cytoplasm and central, round nuclei. Slight pleomorphism may be noted. The interstitial connective tissue strands are delicate (x 100). cf. Figure 15.

Fig. 15. Eccrine hidrocystoma or sudoriferous cyst.

A. (Rec. no. 49, Lab. no. 547/67).
67-year-old man with an elastic skin cyst growing for 2 years. No involvement of the lacrimal punctum. Varying in size. Clinical diagnosis: "cyst of lid".

B. (Rec. no. 210, Lab. no. 546/68).
44-year-old man with multicystic, yellowish tumor for some months. Clinical diagnosis: "cyst of lid".

C and D.
The thin-walled cysts are lined with two rows of flattened epithelial cells. On the skin outside the lids, such cysts originate in sweat ducts. On the lid margin they probably arise from excretory ducts of Moll's glands, although these glands are mainly of apocrine gland origin. Another possibility is origin from ducts of Zeis glands (x 25). cf. Figure 16.

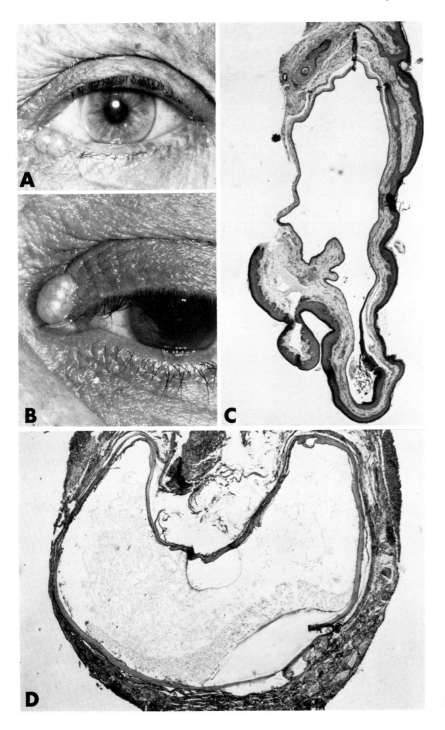

Fig. 15

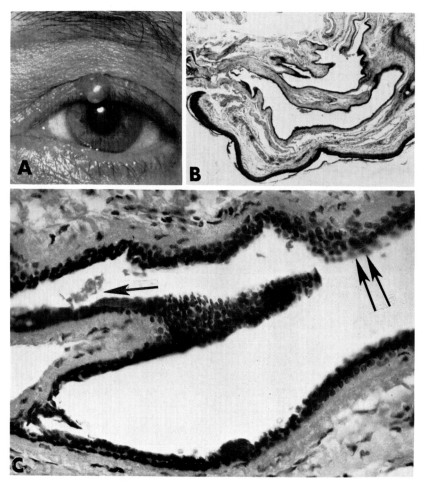

Fig. 16. Apocrine cyst or apocrine hidrocystoma.

A. (Rec. no. 101, Lab. no. 260/66).
   61-year-old woman with a yellowish, smooth tumor for some years. Clinical diagnosis: atheroma.

B. The partially compressed cyst lumen probably has several compartments (x 10).

C. The lining of the lumen shows a row of internal secretory cells *(arrows)* and an external row of cubic cells. Secretory material is seen in the lumen *(arrow)*. It may arise from a blocked excretory duct of a Moll's gland (x 275). cf. Figure 15.

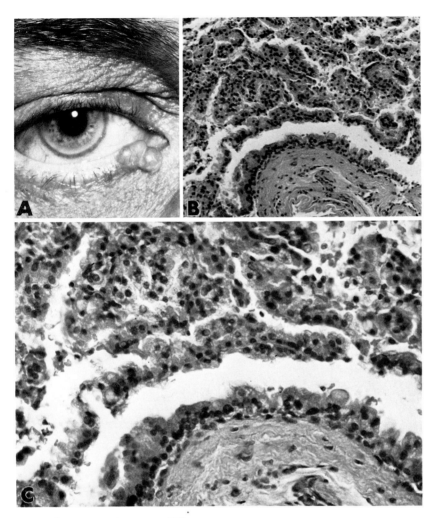

Fig. 17. Syringocystadenoma papilliferum.

A. (Rec. no. 178, Lab. no. 462/66).
   52-year-old man with cystic tumor involving the lacrimal punctum. Growth for some months. Clinical diagnosis: "a cyst."

B. The tumor is composed of villi-like projections into a large lumen (x 25).

C. The projections are lined mainly with two rows of cells, cylindric and cuboidal. They propably originate from apocrine-duct elements (x 275).

Neurogenous Tumors

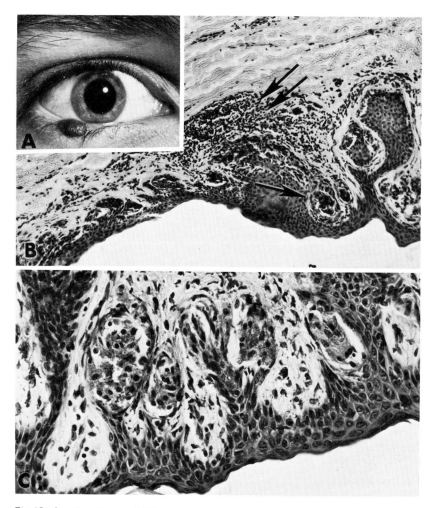

Fig. 18. Junctional nevus of lid.

A. (Rec. no. 149, Lab. no. 636/66).
14-year-old girl with a brown, congenital tumor which has been growing for a few months. Several nevi all over the body. Clinical diagnosis: presumably Recklinghausen's disease.

B. The flat epithelial affection with groups of nevus cells *(arrow)*. The cells in the stroma are lymphocytes *(double arrow)* (x 25).

C. The nevus cells are confined to the epithelium; they are found in epithelial projections toward the stroma (x 275).

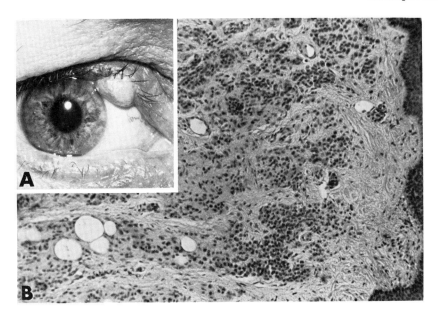

Fig. 19. Intradermal nevus of lid.

A. (Rec. no. 41, Lab. no. 259/67).
   59-year-old woman with a slowly-growing, light tumor, sessile on margin of upper eyelid; it has been growing for 10 years. Clinical diagnosis: papilloma. This is the typical appearance of a nevus falsely diagnosed as papilloma or fibroma.

B. The tumor cells lying in nests in the stroma are separated from the epithelium by a margin of collagen tissue without tumor cells. The epithelium is uninvolved (cf. Fig. 18) (x 100).

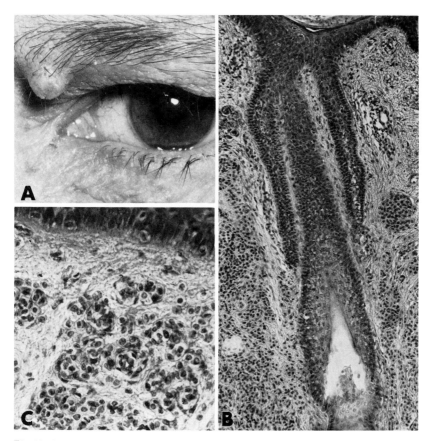

Fig. 20. Intradermal nevus of the supercilium.

A. (Rec. no. 159, Lab. no. 651/68).
   61-year-old woman with initially slowly-growing tumor for many years. Rapid growth for a few months. It was solid, unpigmented, and had a few hairs projecting from the top. Clinical diagnosis: fibroma.

B. Survey of the tumor with sagittally-cut hair surrounded by typical nevus nests (x 25).

C. The intradermal nevus structure is evident (cf. Fig. 19). Projecting hairs are typical of intradermal nevi and are, therefore, a clinical sign of the benign character (x 100).

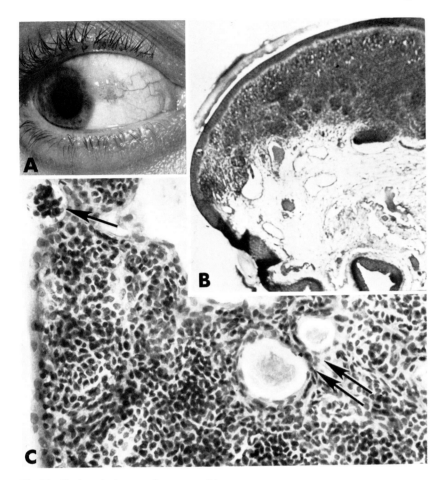

Fig. 21. Conjunctival nevus of compound type.

A. (Rec. no. 218, Lab. no. 497/65).
   18-year-old man with a cystic tumor, unchanged from early childhood. It was slightly pigmented.
   Clinical diagnosis: conjunctival melanosis. These tumors are often completely unpigmented before
   puberty.

B. The subconjunctival tissue is filled with solid tumor tissue with a fairly well-defined border against the
   normal stroma (x 25).

C. The nevus cells are often seen in the atrophic epithelium, frequently as nests *(arrow)*. Small epithelial
   cysts *(double arrow)* in the tumor tissue are characteristic and may be confusing for the pathologist not
   familiar with these conjunctival tumors (x 275).

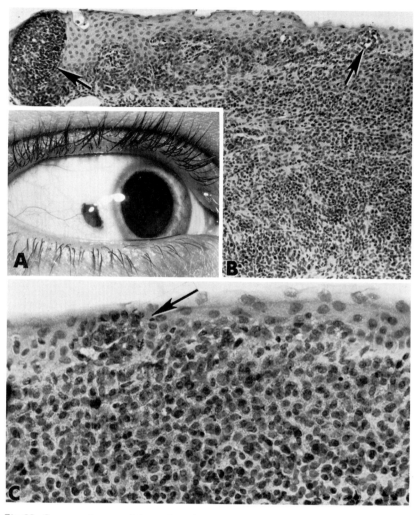

Fig. 22. Compound nevus of the conjunctiva.

A. (Rec. no. 228, Lab. no. 321/67).
   23-year-old man with a dark-brown tumor, growing slightly for 10 years. Clinical diagnosis: conjunctival nevus.

B. The solid tumor tissue is involving the stroma; nests are formed below and subepithelially. Junction activity is seen to the right and left *(arrows)* (x 25).

C. The somewhat atrophic conjunctival epithelium contains nests of nevus cells (junction activity) *(arrow)*. The nevus cells are mostly unpigmented (x 275).

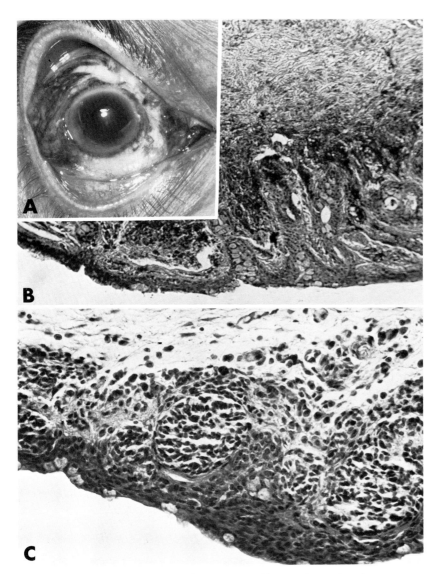

Fig. 23. Recurring compound nevus of conjunctiva with secondary melanosis.

A. (Rec. no. 186, Lab. no. 36/67).
   61-year-old man with a congenital conjunctival nevus. It began to grow when the man was 40 years of age and was then removed totally. Microscopy showed a junctional nevus. Recurrence after 19 years with papillomatous tissue temporally and on the caruncle. Biopsy (Figs. B and C) showed no signs of precancerous melanosis. Observation for 7 years without change.

B. Biopsy from area near caruncle showing a heavy subepithelial melanosis (x 25).

C. Biopsy from temporal papillomatous part showing nevus.cells in the basal part of the epithelium and larger nests subepithelially as well as more diffusely scattered nevus cells in the underlying stroma (x 275).

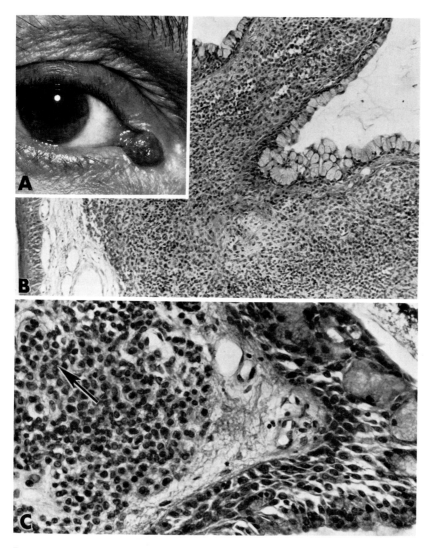

Fig. 24. Nevus of the caruncle (intradermal type).

A. (Rec. no. 223, Lab. no. 45/67).
61-year-old man with unchanged, dark brown, pedunculated, scaling tumor for 20 to 30 years. Clinical diagnosis: nevus of the caruncle.

B. The caruncle tissue is occupied by a solid uniform-celled tissue. Many goblet cells are seen on the surface (x 25).

C. The cells with chromatin-rich nuclei lie diffusely or in small nests *(arrow)* (x 275).

Vascular Tumors

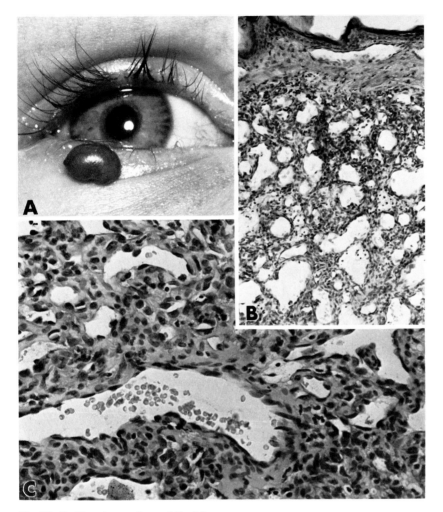

Fig. 25. Capillary hemangioma of the lid.

A. (Rec. no. 273, Lab. no. 33/67).
Two-year-old boy with red, smooth tumor near lower margin for 1 1/2 months. Started as a pinpoint affection. Rapid growth. Clinical diagnosis: hemangioma.

B. The lesion is composed of proliferating endothelial cells forming uniform lumina. Inflammation is slight or absent. The so-called "hemangioma" of granulation tissue type (pyogenic granuloma) has the same morphology, but leukocyte infiltration is heavy (x 25).

C. The vascular spaces are lined with flat endothelial cells. Later, fibrosis may appear which then leads to shrinkage and clinical healing (x 275).

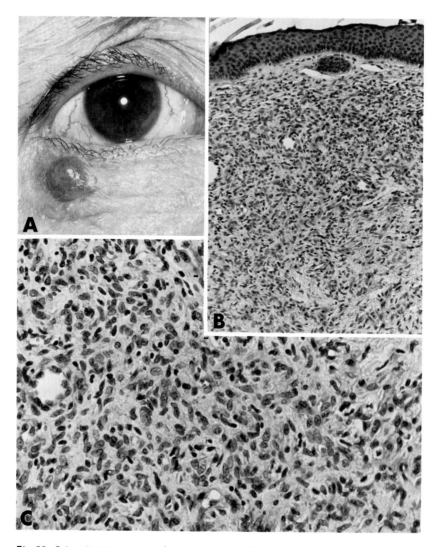

Fig. 26. Sclerosing hemangioma (dermatofibroma, fibrous histiocytoma. Different terms may be used, depending upon the amount of fibroblasts, histiocytes and/or capillaries).

A. (Rec. no. 133, Lab. no. 184/67).
   49-year-old woman with a bluish tumor for 1 year. Not compressible or pulsating. Clinical diagnosis: hemangioma.

B. The tumor is solid with abundant fibrosis and only few vascular lumina. The fairly uniform picture is apparent (x 25).

C. The cells are spindle-shaped with tapered ends; collagen fibrils proceed from the ends and fill the inter-cellular space. The chromatin content varies. A single nucleolus is often seen (x 275).

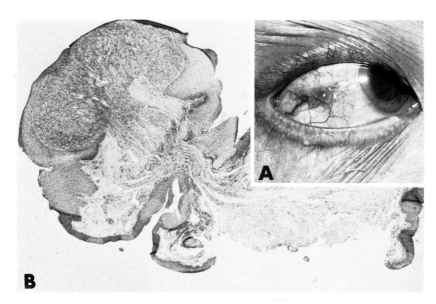

Fig. 27. Capillary hemangioma of conjunctiva.

A. (Rec. no. 189, Lab. no. 225/66).
   69-year-old man with a cystic conjunctival tumor for years. Numerous vessels leading to the tumor can be seen. Clinical diagnosis: aneurysm.

B. Survey of the lesion composed of fairly solid proliferating endothelial cells (x 10). The morphology is similar to Figure 25. A pyogenic granuloma (or "hemangioma" of the granulation tissue type) has the same structure; but in addition, a pronounced amount of inflammatory cells, predominantly neutrophilic leukocytes.

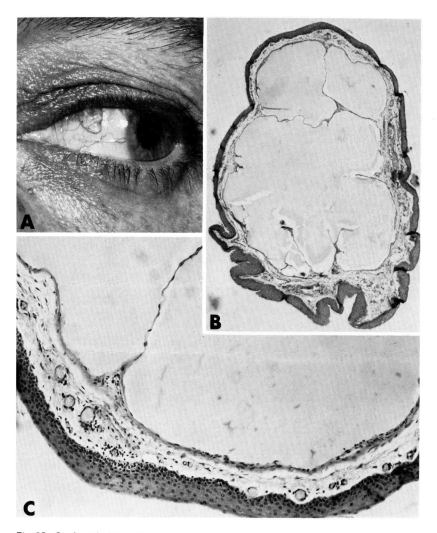

Fig. 28. Conjunctival lymphangioma.

A. (Rec. no. 97, Lab. no. 491/65).
   44-year-old woman with a multicystic conjunctival tumor for 1 year. Several vessels leading to the cyst.
   Clinical diagnosis: conjunctival cyst.

B. The cyst is well-defined and is divided into several compartments by thin strands of connective tissue
   (× 10).

C. The wall is composed of a connective tissue with a few vessels and is lined with flat endothelium. The
   conjunctival epithelium on the outside contains no goblet cells (× 100).

Mesodermal Soft Tissue Tumors

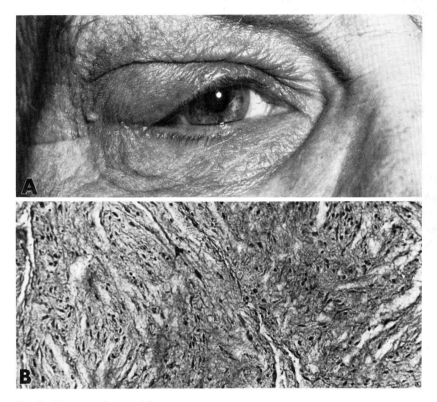

Fig. 29. Myxoma of upper lid.

A. (Rec. no. 138, Lab. no. 134/68).
65-year-old man with an indolent tumor for 4 to 5 months. Slow growth. Normal skin above the tumor.
Clinical diagnosis: ectopic lacrimal gland.
cf. Figures 31 and 32.

B. This benign tumor is composed of spindle-shaped or stellate fibroblasts. The stroma is mucinous and replaces the normal dermal collagen. It stains positively with alcian blue and metachromatically with toluidine blue. It is hyaluronidase sensitive (x 100).

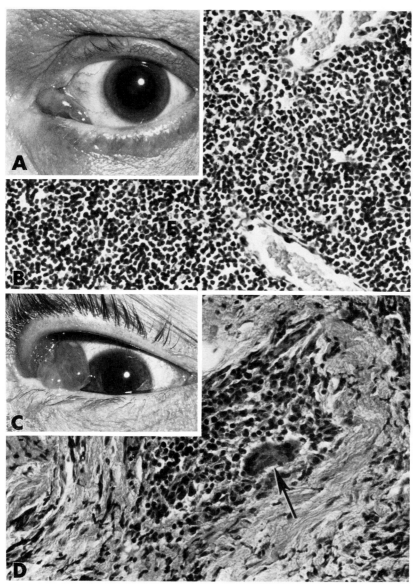

Fig. 30. Conjunctival lymphocytic infiltration (lymphoid lesion of undeterminate nature) compared with a hypertrophic chalazion.

A. (Rec. no. 284, Lab. no. 314/66). 56-year-old man with a rapidly-growing conjunctival tumor for 1 year. The tumor was transparent and solid. No general manifestations after 8 years.

B. The dense uniform lymphocytic infiltration in the subconjunctival tissue. Such an infiltration may be a forerunner of a systemic disease such as lymphosarcoma. It may also be seen as an immunologic reaction. Presence of conjunctival and orbital lymphocytic infiltrations may even be seen in the event of a malignant tumor elsewhere (e.g., broncial carcinoma). They always indicate the necessity for thorough general examination and observation (x 275).

C. (Rec. no. 220, Lab. no. 393/67). 23-year-old man had the tumor shown for 1 month. The similar clinical appearance of this tumor and the tumor of Figure 30 A is evident.

D. Typical chalazion tissue with a giant cell *(arrow)* and lymphocytes (cf. Color Plate IV G and H) (x 275).

Fig. 31. Dermoid cysts. ▶

A. (Rec. no. 11, Lab. no. 157/68). 16-year-old boy with a cyst lateral in the superciliary region. The cyst has been present since the boy was 2 years old. The overlying skin was normal. The cyst was freely movable against the base, but varied in size. This is the typical localization (cf. Figs. 29 and 32).

B. (Rec. no. 294, Lab. no. 172/66b). 19-year-old woman with tumor for many years. Constant in size and freely movable. This is an atypical localization for a dermoid cyst.

C. Survey of the fairly thin cyst wall. The structure is similar in both cases (x 10).

D. The wall is composed of stratified squamous epithelium. In the lumen *(below)*, keratin lamellas are abundant. A sharp shift to granulation tissue *(right)* is to be seen (x 100).

E. Survey of the compressed cyst. Sebaceous glands are to be seen in the wall *(arrow)* (x 40).

F. Strong foreign-body reaction in the wall. A cut hair is to be seen in the lumen *(arrow)* (x 100).

Choristomas

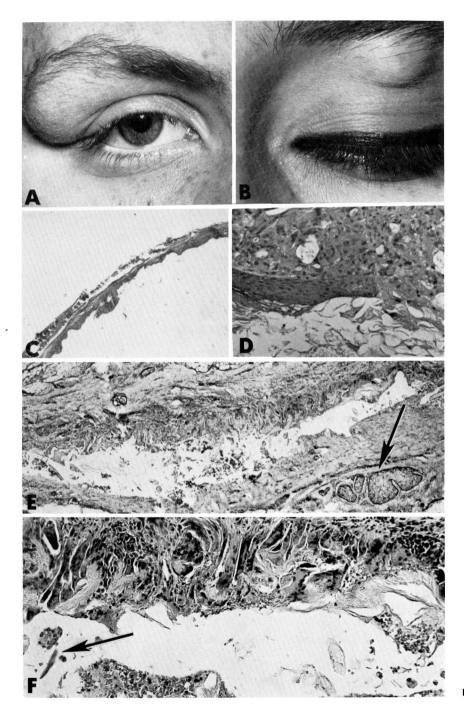

Fig. 31

Miscellaneous

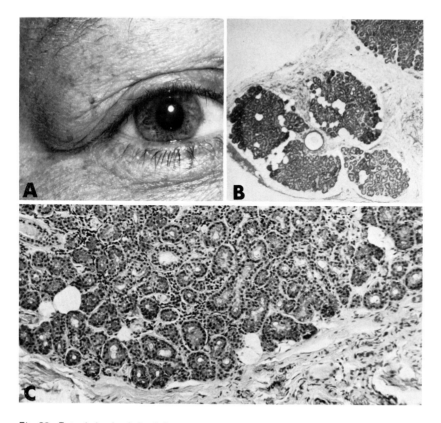

Fig. 32. Ectopic lacrimal gland tissue.

A. (Rec. no. 143, Lab. no. 496/67).
   42-year-old woman with tumor lateral in upper lid for 4 to 5 years, soft and cystic on the conjunctival side, can be compressed into orbit. Clinical diagnosis: "duct cyst." cf. Figures 29 and 31.

B. The tumor is composed of lobules of glandular tissue divided by connective tissue strands (x 10).

C. The characteristic lacrimal gland tissue of normal appearance (x 100).

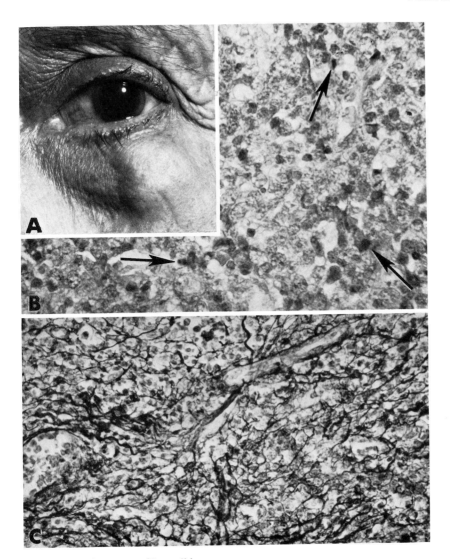

Fig. 33. Reticulosarcoma of lower lid.

A. (Rec. no. 251, Lab. no. 565/66).
   59-year-old woman with a rapidly-growing tumor for 1 month without symptoms. The tumor was movable in relation to the skin and the base. No lesions in any other organ. "Sarcoma". Radiation therapy. Bilateral choroidal reticulosarcoma 5 years later. Patient died 6 years later of cerebral involvement.

B. The tumor is composed of large pleomorphic reticulum cells placed closely together. Several cells have a light cytoplasm. Mitoses are abundant *(arrows)* (x 275).

C. The reticulum staining is positive. Numerous reticular fibres are often seen around single cells (x 100).

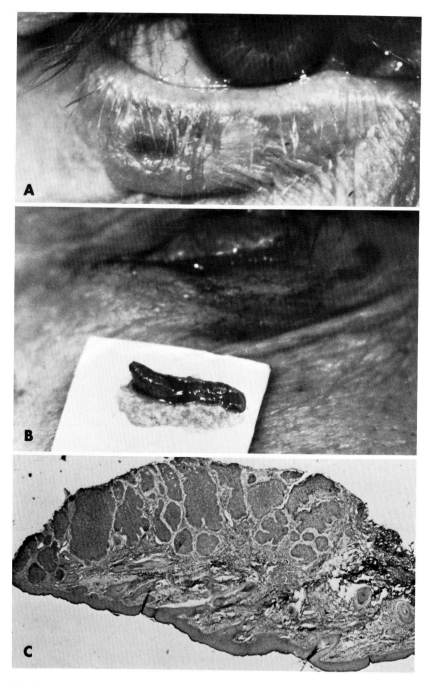

Fig. 34. Open marginal biopsy.

A. Typical basal cell carcinoma (rodent ulcer) of lower eyelid.

B. The tumor area is outlined with ink. The marginal biopsy has been performed. The slice of tissue including normal skin is placed on the cardboard. The wound edges are nearly agglutinated.

C. Survey of the biopsy. Normal tissue to the right. The skin surface is below. Tumor tissue is seen upward and to the left; it corresponds to the bottom and central part of the tumor.

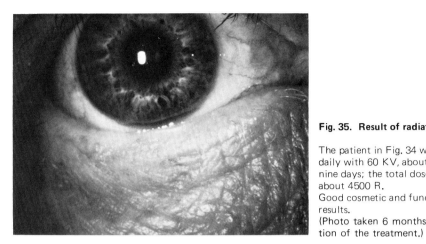

Fig. 35. Result of radiation therapy.

The patient in Fig. 34 was treated
daily with 60 KV, about 500 R for
nine days; the total dose thus was
about 4500 R.
Good cosmetic and functional
results.
(Photo taken 6 months after termina-
tion of the treatment.)

Recommended Literature

1. Andersen, S. Ry: Radiotherapy of eye diseases. Trans. Pac. Coast Oto-Ophthal. Soc. (1969) 237–263.
2. Aurora, A. L., F. C. Blodi: Lesions of the eyelids: A clinicopathological study. Survey of Ophthal. 15 (1970) 94–104.
3. Boniuk, M.: Tumors of the eyelids. In: Tumors of the eye and adnexa. International ophthalmology clinics, vol. 2/2, L. E. Zimmermann, Ed. Little, Brown and Co., Boston 1962.
4. Duke-Elder, S., P. A. MacFaul: The ocular adnexa. System of ophthalmology, vol. VIII/1. Henry Kingston, London 1974.
5. Enzinger, F. M., R. Lattes, H. Torloni: Histological typing of soft tissue tumours. International classification of tumors, No. 3. WHO, Geneva 1969.
6. Greer, C. H.: Ocular pathology. 2nd ed. Blackwell Scientific Publications, Oxford, London, Edinburgh and Melbourne 1972.
7. Halnan, K. E., M. J. H. Britten: Late functional and cosmetic results of treatment of eyelid tumors. Brit. J. Ophthal. 52 (1968) 43–53.
8. Hogan, M. J., L. E. Zimmermann: Ophthalmic pathology. An atlas and textbook. 2nd ed. W. B. Saunders Co., Philadelphia and London 1962.
9. Leventhal, H. H., R. J. Messer: Malignant tumors of the eyelid. Amer. J. Surg. 124 (1972) 522–526.
10. Lever, W. F.: Histopathology of the skin. 4th ed. Pitman Medical Publishing Co., Ltd., London 1967.
11. Lund, H. Z.: Tumors of the skin. Atlas of tumor pathology. Sect. I/Fasc. 2. Armed Forces Institute of Pathology, Washington, D.C. 1957 – .
12. Montgomery, H.: Dermatopathology, vols. I and II. Hoeber Medical Division. Harper & Row Publishers, New York, Evanston, and London 1967.
13. Offret, G., P. Dhermy, A. Brini, P. Bec: Anatomie pathologique de l'oeil et de ses annexes. Masson & Cie., Paris 1974.
14. Reese, A. B.: Tumors of the eye. 2nd ed. Hoeber Medical Division. Harper & Row Publishers, New York, Evanston and London 1963.
15. Ten Seldam, R. E. J., E. B. Helwig, L. H. Sobin, H. Torloni: Histological typing of skin tumours. International classification of tumors No. 12, WHO, Geneva 1974.
16. Yanoff, M., B. S. Fine: Ocular pathology. A text and atlas. Harper & Row Ltd., London 1975.

Glossary

(*Italics* indicate that the term is listed separately)

Acanthosis *Hyperplasia* and/or hypertrophy of the prickle-cell layer (stratum Malpighii) of the skin. The prickle-cell layer is the layer lying immediately above the basal layer. The polygonal cells are united into a mosaic by intercellular bridges. A. is seen in keratoacanthomas and several skin diseases, e.g., a. nigricans.

Actinic rays Rays of light, especially of the longer-wave part of the spectrum, producing chemical and biological effects, e.g., on the skin.

Adenoma A benign epithelial tumor composed of glandular or gland-like elements, usually originating in glandular tissue, e.g., *sebaceous adenoma* of sebaceous glands (Fig. 12).

Adnexal structures The appendages of the lids, i.e., hair follicles, *glands of Meibom,* (modified sebaceous glands), sebaceous glands of Zeis and ciliary sweat glands of Moll.

Adnexal tumors Benign or malignant tumors with origin in *adnexal structures.*

Appendages, dermal See adnexal structures.

Apocrine cyst See Moll cyst.

Atheroma See epidermal and sebaceous cysts.

Basal cell carcinoma (Basal cell epithelioma, basalioma, rodent ulcer.) Malignant epithelial tumor of the skin consisting of cells resembling the basal cells of the epidermis but without intercellular bridges. Horn cysts may be found. The periorbital region is the most common location. The tumors do not metastasize but grow invasively, a serious complication when they grow into the facial bones. Many theories of origin (Figs. 7, 8, 9).

Basal cell papilloma (Seborrheic keratosis, verruca senilis.) A benign skin tumor consisting of basal cells like the basal cells of the epidermis; intercellular bridges together with *acanthosis* and hyperkeratosis are found, usually only with slight papillomatosis. Cysts containing keratin lamellas are found in the solid strands (Fig. 2).

Calcifying epithelioma of Malherbe See pilomatrixoma.

Caruncle Also lacrimal caruncle. The small eminence medially in the conjunctiva. It contains sebaceous glands and small hairs and is covered by conjunctival epithelium. Together with the plica semilunaris, it is considered an atavistic structure corresponding to the nictitating membrane of animals.

Chalazion A granulomatous inflammation of the lid induced by sebum from distended meibomian glands (lipogranuloma). It consists of epithelioid cells, foreign body giant cells around fat vacuoles, lymphocytes, and eosinophils (Fig. 30; Color Plate IV G, H).

Choristoma A tumor consisting of tissue which is normally not found at the site concerned. A dermoid cyst is a c. (Fig. 31). In contrast, a hamartoma only involves tissue elements normally found at the site concerned.

Complex nevus See intradermal nevus.

Compound nevus A tumor of *nevus* cells. It consists of nests of nevus cells located within the (basal part of the) epidermis (junction activity) in contact with the epidermis (dropping off) and of cells in the dermis without contact with the epidermis (Figs. 21, 22).

Cyst Usually a spherical well-defined lesion, often with an epithelial lining and containing a liquid or semi-solid material, e.g., *epidermal, sebaceous, conjunctival cyst.*

Dermal appendages See adnexal structures.

Dermoid cyst A *choristoma* due to inclusion of foreign tissue, possibly in the closure of a developmental cleft. It has a lining of epidermis and a connective tissue wall with rudimentary sebaceous glands, sweat glands and hair follicles, and is filled with keratin lamellas, sebaceous material, and fragments of hairs. The superciliary region is the most frequent location in the skin (Fig. 31).

Eccrine hidrocystoma See Moll cyst.

Ectopic tissue Tissue of normal structure located away from normal position, e.g., e. lacrimal gland tissue in the lower lid.

Epidermal tumor Tumor consisting of epidermal elements.

Epidermal cyst Intracutaneous or subcutaneous *cyst* with a lining of epidermis and filled with keratin lamellas but without *adnexal structures* in the wall (cf. dermoid cyst). Clinically indistinguishable from *sebaceous cyst.* E.c. appears as "atheroma" (Fig. 4, 5).

Epithelial cyst Cyst from epithelial structures, e.g., conjunctival cyst.

Fibroma A benign mesodermal tumor usually composed of fully developed connective tissue.

Foreign body granuloma A *granuloma* formed as a response to a foreign material not tolerated by the surrounding tissue (e.g., a suture granuloma).

Granulation tissue Small fleshy masses of tissue formed in wounds; composed of proliferating capillaries and fibroblasts; often contains neutrophilic leukocytes (pyogenic g.t.).

Granuloma A tumor or nodule with a variety of structures, usually of an inflammatory nature. In pathology, the word is usually used for an epithelioid cell granuloma consisting of epithelioid cells (derived from histiocytes); sometimes forms giant cells and is surrounded by lymphocytes. The center of the g. may be necrotic as in tuberculosis. See *foreign body g.* and *chalazion.*

Hemangioma A congenital benign tumor consisting of a glomerulus of vessels. Capillary, arteriovenous and cavernous h. are the most usual types (Figs. 25, 27; Color Plate III F, G, H).

Hemangioendothelioma A vascular tumor consisting of proliferating endothelial cells forming numerous small vascular tubes surrounded by more cells than required to line the lumina with a single endothelial layer. These tumors have malignant potentialities, but seldom recur when properly removed. Malignant signs are: pleomorphic, atypical, or anaplastic endothelial cells with more mitoses proliferating into the lumina of the tubes; the lumina are obscured and the regular pattern distorted (malignant h. or hemangioendotheliosarcoma) (Color Plate III D).

Hematoma A tumor-like enlargement produced in the tissue by escaped blood (a hemorrhage). If not resorbed, it will be transformed by fibroblasts into an organized h.; a fibrous nodule is formed.

Hyperplasia Abnormal increase in number of normal cells (in contrast to hypertrophy which is due to an enlargement of the single cells), e.g., h. of sebaceous or *meibomian glands.*

Intradermal nevus A benign tumor composed of *nevus cells* and nests and/or columns of nevus cells located in the dermis and separated from each other and from the epidermis by dermal connective tissue. The nevus cells may form groups around hair follicles (Figs. 19, 20, 24; Color Plate IV A, B, C). In the lower dermis, curled structures resembling Meissner tactile corpuscles, may sometimes be observed, a neuronevus, or nevus complexus (cf. compound n.) (Color Plate IV D, E, F).

Junctional nevus (Superficial n.). A group of nevus cells lying in the basal part of the epidermis and at the epidermodermal junction. It is the type of nevus that is most often the origin of a malignant melanoma of the skin (Fig. 18).

Keratoacanthoma A benign tumor most frequent in the face and at the back of the hands. Rapid growth (a history of a few months) and tendency to spontaneous regression are typical. A central keratin plug is seen in a cup-like invagination of the epidermis showing *acanthosis,* keratosis, and irregular proliferations into the dermis, sometimes making differentiation from squamous cell carcinoma difficult (Color Plate I D, E, F).

Keratotic papilloma (Squamous cell papilloma). A benign tumor consisting of one or more papillary projections with a connective tissue core covered by a cornified, stratified squamous epithelium which produces an abundance of keratin. It may be pigmented. Some have viral etiology. (Fig. 1; Color Plate I A, B, C).

Leukoplakia (Leukokeratosis). A grayish-white, plate-like, slightly elevated patch on a surface, most often a mucous membrane. It is a clinical term. Histopathologically, hyperkeratosis, atypical epidermal cells and a heavy inflammatory infiltrate are found.

Lymphangioma A benign, possibly congenital, tumor composed of distended lymph vessels containing coagulated lymph, lymphocytes, and occasionally erythrocytes (Fig. 28).

Lymphoma (Lymphoid lesion of undeterminate nature). A tumor-like lesion composed almost exclusively of lymphocytes; most often mature in the orbital region. A lymphoma may be an immunological manifestation or the initial phase of or a part of a lymphatic leukemia or lymphosarcoma (malignant lymphoma). The history and the clinical examination are decisive; frequently only the subsequent history reveals the nature (Fig. 30).

Meibomian carcinoma (Sebaceous carcinoma). A malignant epithelial tumor originating in the *meibomian glands.* It consists of irregular lobular formations of undifferentiated sebaceous cells. This tumor may be so anaplastic that it is difficult to distinguish from a basal cell carcinoma, but it is more malignant than this tumor (Color Plate III A, B, C).

Meibomian glands Modified sebaceous glands of the tarsus.

Melanosis An increased number of melanocytes or an increased melanin content in a normal number of melanocytes in the skin or conjunctiva. cf. precancerous m.

Melanocyte A cell derived from the neural crest, synthesizing the specialized melanin-containing organelle, the melanosome. M. are normally found in the epidermis, dermis, and uveal tract of the eye. On rare occasions, they are found in man in mucous membranes, including the conjunctiva.

Melanoma A tumor composed of cells capable of forming melanosomes (cf. melanocyte) with absent, partial or complete melanization. M. may be amelanotic or melanotic, benign or malignant.

Mesodermal soft tissue tumor See soft tissue tumor.

Moll cyst (Eccrine hidrocystoma, apocrine hidrocystoma, sudoriferous cyst). A Moll cyst is formed by a blocked excretory duct from a Moll's gland (see *adnexal structures*) lined by two or more layers of flat or cuboidal cells. It is indistinguishable from a sudoriferous cyst from the duct of a sweat gland on the skin. Apocrine secretion may be demonstrated in some (Figs. 15, 16).

Molluscum contagiosum Small, soft, virus-induced, rounded tumors of the skin with a central depression (umbo). Most frequent in the face. Histopathologically, the epidermis grows down into the dermis and the epidermal cells are changed by cytoplasmic inclusion bodies, the so-called molluscum bodies, which displace and compress the nucleus of the epidermal cell. The inclusion body increases in size from the basal layer toward the surface, where the cells burst and empty their viral content.

Myxoma A benign, mesodermal, soft tissue tumor composed of undifferentiated fibroblasts with the ability of the embryonal fibroblast to produce mucin (Fig. 29).

Nevus In this work, synonymous with pigmented or melanocytic nevus. A benign, neuroectodermal tumor composed of nevus cells or *melanocytes.* The typical nevus cell is oval or cuboidal with somewhat light, slightly eosinophilic cytoplasm and round to oval, somewhat chromatin-rich nucleus (cf. junctional, compound, and intradermal nevus).

Neurogenous tumor (Neuroectodermal t.). A tumor arising in elements derived from the nervous system. Primarily a clinical term.

Neuronaevus See intradermal nevus.

Papilloma A benign, branching tumor derived from epithelium (cf. keratotic p.).

Parakeratinization An imperfect keratinization resulting in retention of nuclei in the horny layer. Often seen in areas with metaplasia (change of one type of tissue into another) of cuboidal into stratified squamous epithelium.

Pilomatrixoma (Benign calcifying epithelioma of Malherbe). Most frequent in the face. It is composed of masses of epidermal cells surrounded by connective tissue of the dermis. In addition to viable epidermal cells, necrotic epidermal cells, so-called shadow cells, are encountered, sometimes with calcifications (Color Plate I G, H).

Precancerous lesion A lesion which according to experience and morphology will eventually become malignant.

Precancerous melanosis A *melanosis* (involving the conjunctiva) which eventually transforms into a malignant melanoma. Histopathologically, it is a diffuse *junctional nevus.*

Reticulosarcoma (Reticulum cell sarcoma). A highly malignant tumor often typically seen in the lymph nodes but also occurring in many other locations, e.g., the skin. It is composed of large pleomorphic reticulum cells with abundant cytoplasm and large nuclei. The reticulin content is usually high (Fig. 33).

Rodent ulcer See basal cell carcinoma.

Schwannoma (Neurinoma, neurilemmona). A well-defined, benign tumor around or in relation to a nerve. It is composed of spindle-shaped, fibril-producing cells in intercrossing columns. The nuclei are often arranged at the same level; a palisade-like pattern is produced. Malignant schwannomas are rare.

Sclerosing hemangioma (Dermatofibroma, histiocytoma). A tumor composed of fibroblasts, collagen, histiocytes and capillaries. The term is often adapted to the dominant cells: fibroblasts in dermatofibroma, histiocytes in histiocytoma, endothelial cells forming capillaries or capillaries in regressive fibrosis in s.h. (Fig. 26).

Sebaceous adenoma An *adenoma* composed of sebaceous cells with a clear, slightly granulated cytoplasm and a central, rather small, vesicular nucleus. In the lids, it often originates from the *meibomian glands* (Fig. 12; Color Plate II F, G, H).

Sebaceous carcinoma See meibomian carcinoma.

Sebaceous cyst A *cyst* from *adnexal,* immature *structures.* The cyst is lined by epithelial cells (often vacuolated) simulating sebaceous cells; it is filled with disintegrated cells. More or less epidermal differentiation may occur. See also epidermal cyst.

Seborrheic keratosis See basal cell papilloma.

Soft tissue tumor A tumor originating in the soft tissues of the body, i.e., all nonepithelial, extraskeletal tissues. The reticuloendothelial system is excluded.

Squamous cell carcinoma A malignant tumor of skin and mucous membranes. It is invasive and, in contrast to the basal cell carcinoma, metastasizes, primarily to the lymph nodes. It is composed of irregular strands and islands of more or less undifferentiated epidermal cells; it proliferates downward into the dermis. Differentiation is in the direction of keratinization; it appears as horn pearls (Figs. 10, 11).

Squamous cell papilloma See keratotic papilloma.

Sudoriferous cyst See Moll cyst.

Syringocystadenoma (Papillary syringocystadenoma, syringocystadenoma papilliferum).

A benign tumor with differentiation toward apocrine ducts; it is composed of cystic spaces with villi-like projections extending into the lumina. These are lined with two rows of cuboidal cells; the most peripheral of these cells are immature myoepithelial cells (Fig. 17).

Xanthelasma A group of neutral fat-laden histiocytes in the dermis of the eyelids. Relation to hypercholesterolemia is rare.

Subject Index

(Page numbers in *italics* refer to the histopathological section)